Table of Contents

1 Introduction

3 Common Health Concerns
Learn more about the medical concerns you might have

4	Arthritis Advice
9	Cancer Facts for People Over 50
13	Depression: Don't Let the Blues Hang Around
18	Diabetes in Older People—A Disease You Can Manage
22	Forgetfulness: It's Not Always What You Think
26	Hearing Loss
30	High Blood Pressure
33	HIV, AIDS, and Older People
38	Menopause
44	Osteoporosis: The Bone Thief
49	Prostate Problems
53	Shingles
57	Stroke
60	Urinary Incontinence

65 Staying Healthy
How to keep your body working well

66	A Good Night's Sleep
69	Aging and Your Eyes
73	Alcohol Use and Abuse
76	Concerned About Constipation?
79	Dietary Supplements: More is Not Always Better
84	Exercise: Getting Fit for Life
88	Foot Care

91	*Good Nutrition: It's a Way of Life*
98	*Life Extension: Science Fact or Science Fiction?*
104	*Sexuality in Later Life*
109	*Shots for Safety*
114	*Skin Care and Aging*
120	*Smoking: It's Never Too Late to Stop*
125	*Taking Care of Your Teeth and Mouth*
129	*What to Do About Flu*

133 Getting Good Health Care
What to remember when you need medical help

134	*Choosing a Doctor*
139	*Considering Surgery?*
142	*Health Quackery: Spotting Health Scams*
145	*Hospital Hints*
150	*Medicines: Use Them Safely*
153	*Online Health Information: Can You Trust It?*

157 Staying Safe and Planning Ahead
How to protect yourself now and plan for the future

158	*Crime and Older People*
162	*Getting Your Affairs in Order*
166	*Hyperthermia—Too Hot for Your Health*
170	*Hypothermia: A Cold Weather Hazard*
175	*Long-Term Care: Choosing the Right Place*
180	*Older Drivers*
184	*Preventing Falls and Fractures*

187 Appendix
Tips from the National Institute on Aging

188	*There's No Place Like Home—For Growing Old*
194	*Understanding Risk: What Do Those Headlines Really Mean?*
198	*Alzheimer's Disease*

204 Index

Introduction

Alan and Ken have been good friends and neighbors in their small town for 40 years. Their lives are very similar. They work in the same office. They help each other with chores like shoveling their snow-covered driveways. Each of their wives keeps an eye on her husband's health, too. Although they both felt fine, today Alan and Ken each went to the doctor for a checkup because their wives suggested it was time. They were each surprised to find out about a new medical problem. Now, they each want more information about their health, and that's where their stories start being different. Alan doesn't know where to start; Ken knows exactly where to look.

The doctor surprised Alan with the news that he has high blood pressure and took a few minutes to explain the problem. When she asked if he had any questions, Alan said no. So, the doctor gave him a prescription for medicine to lower his high blood pressure, and Alan left. By the time he got home, however, Alan realized there were other things he wanted to know about his condition, but he didn't know where to look. And, he thought, I feel fine—why bother to take another pill?

Ken also didn't expect to be told he has high blood pressure. Just like Alan, at first the doctor's explanation was enough for Ken. He took his prescription for medicine and headed home. But on his way home, Ken, too, thought of more questions. So, he went to the bookcase in the living room and took out a book his wife just got from the National Institute on Aging. Sure enough, in *Bound for Your Good Health: A Collection of Age Pages*, Ken found a section explaining high blood pressure. It even had places to contact for more information. Ken was able to get answers to his questions. He learned how important it is to take his medicine just like the doctor ordered.

More Information About This Book

Bound for Your Good Health is a good place to start finding information on a wide range of subjects. Right at your fingertips are *Age Pages* on many familiar medical problems, as well as on other health matters of interest to older people. *Age Pages* from the National Institute on Aging (NIA), part of the National Institutes of Health, are fact sheets written about a variety of health subjects related to growing older. People have been using *Age Pages* for more than two decades to get accurate answers to common health questions. You may have come across an *Age Page* in your doctor's office or at the local library. Maybe you read about them in the newspaper. Or, possibly, you called or wrote the NIA with a question about a health problem and got an *Age Page* as part of the answer.

The *Age Pages* are so popular because they are easy-to-read, answer basic questions, and suggest other resources where the reader can learn more. People know they can depend on what they read in these because the information comes from scientific research.

This collection brings all the *Age Pages* together to make it easier for you to find the information you need. In addition, the *Age Pages* are organized into chapters that give you a broad look at different types of subjects. Finally, an in-depth index can help you pinpoint the exact information you need quickly and accurately. And, don't miss the bonus tip sheets included in the Appendix at the back.

Bound for Your Good Health gives you a starting point to answer most of your basic questions about your health as you grow older. In it, you may also discover new ways to take good care of yourself, as well as many helpful resources. We have tried to make sure that all information is up-to-date. But remember that medical research is ongoing—experts are always learning new things about aging and disease. The date at the end of each *Age Page* lets you know when the information was last reviewed by NIA's experts. Please note that organizations often move or change their phone numbers, so, in a few cases, by the time you read this, some of the resources may have changed. For the very latest on these topics, you can call 800-222-2225 or go online to *www.niapublications.org*, the NIA's publications website.

By the way, wondering whether Alan ever found answers to his questions about high blood pressure? Alan and his wife now have their own copy of *Bound for Your Good Health*. When Ken learned about Alan's problems getting answers to his questions, he gave Alan the toll-free number to call for his own free copy.

Common Health Concerns

Learn more about the medical concerns you might have

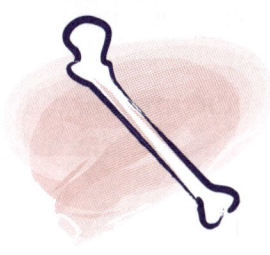

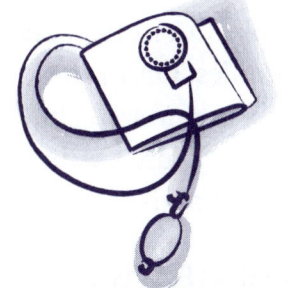

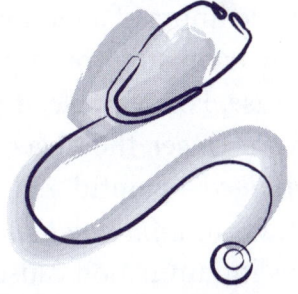

4	Arthritis Advice
9	Cancer Facts for People Over 50
13	Depression: Don't Let the Blues Hang Around
18	Diabetes in Older People—A Disease You Can Manage
22	Forgetfulness: It's Not Always What You Think
26	Hearing Loss
30	High Blood Pressure
33	HIV, AIDS, and Older People
38	Menopause
44	Osteoporosis: The Bone Thief
49	Prostate Problems
53	Shingles
57	Stroke
60	Urinary Incontinence

Arthritis Advice

"Arthritis" is not just a word doctors use when they talk about painful, stiff joints. In fact, there are many kinds of arthritis, each with different symptoms and treatments. Most types of arthritis are chronic. That means they can go on for a long period of time.

Arthritis can attack joints in almost any part of the body. Some forms of arthritis cause changes you can see and feel—swelling, warmth, and redness in your joints. In some the pain and swelling last only a short time, but are very bad. Other types cause less troublesome symptoms, but still slowly damage your joints.

Common Kinds of Arthritis

Arthritis is one of the most common diseases in this country. Millions of adults and half of all people age 65 and older are troubled by this disease. Older people most often have osteoarthritis, rheumatoid arthritis, or gout.

Osteoarthritis (OA) is the most common type of arthritis in older people. OA starts when cartilage begins to become ragged and wears away. Cartilage is the tissue that pads bones in a joint. At OA's worst, all of the cartilage in a joint wears away, leaving bones that rub against each other. You are most likely to have OA in your hands, neck, lower back, or the large weight-bearing joints of your body, such as knees and hips.

OA symptoms can range from stiffness and mild pain that comes and goes with activities like walking, bending, or stooping to severe joint pain that keeps on even when you rest or try to sleep. Sometimes OA causes your joints to feel stiff when you haven't moved them in a while, like after riding in the car. But the stiffness goes away when you move the joint. In time OA can also cause problems moving joints and sometimes disability if your back, knees, or hips are affected.

What causes OA? Growing older is what most often puts you at risk for OA. Other than that, scientists think the cause depends on which part of the body is involved. For example, OA in the hands or hips may run in families. OA in the knees can be linked with being overweight. Injuries or overuse may cause OA in joints such as knees, hips, or hands.

Rheumatoid Arthritis (RA) is an *autoimmune* disease. In RA, that means your body attacks the lining of a joint just as it would if it were trying to protect you from injury or disease. For example, if you had a splinter in your finger, the finger would become *inflamed*—painful, red, and swollen. RA leads to *inflammation* in your joints. This inflammation causes pain, swelling, and stiffness that lasts for hours. This can often happen in many different joints at the same time. You might not even be able to move the joint. People with RA often don't feel well. They may be tired or run a fever. People of any age can develop RA, and it is more common in women.

RA can attack almost any joint in the body, including the joints in the fingers, wrists, shoulders, elbows, hips, knees, ankles, feet, and neck. If you have RA in a joint on one side of the body, the same joint on the other side of your body will probably have RA also. RA not only destroys joints. It can also attack organs such as the heart, muscles, blood vessels, nervous system, and eyes.

Gout is one of the most painful forms of arthritis. An attack can begin when crystals of uric acid form in the connective tissue and/or joint spaces. These deposits lead to swelling, redness, heat, pain, and stiffness in the joint. Gout attacks often follow eating foods like shellfish, liver, dried beans, peas, anchovies, or gravy. Using alcohol, being overweight, and certain medications may also make gout worse. In older people, some blood pressure medicines can also increase your chance of a gout attack.

Gout is most often a problem in the big toe, but it can affect other joints, including your ankle, elbow, knee, wrist, hand, or other toes. Swelling may cause the skin to pull tightly around the joint and make the area red or purple and very tender. Your doctor might suggest blood tests and x-rays. He or she might also take a sample of fluid from your joint while you are having an attack.

Other forms of arthritis include psoriatic arthritis (in people with the skin condition psoriasis), ankylosing spondylitis (which mostly affects the spine), reactive arthritis (arthritis that occurs as a reaction to another illness in the body), and arthritis in the temporomandibular joint (where the jaw joins the skull).

Warning Signs

You might have some form of arthritis if you have:

- Lasting joint pain,
- Joint swelling,
- Joint stiffness,
- Tenderness or pain when touching a joint,
- Problems using or moving a joint as normal, or
- Warmth and redness in a joint.

If any one of these symptoms lasts longer than 2 weeks, see your regular doctor or a rheumatologist. If you have a fever, feel physically ill, suddenly have a swollen joint, or have problems using your joint, see your doctor sooner. Your health care provider will ask questions about your symptoms and do a physical exam. He or she may take x-rays or do lab tests before suggesting a treatment plan.

Treating Arthritis

Each kind of arthritis is handled a little differently, but there are some common treatment choices. Rest, exercise, eating a healthy, well-balanced diet, and learning the right way to use and protect your joints are key to living with any kind of arthritis. The right shoes and a cane can help with pain in the feet, knees, and hips when walking. You can also find gadgets to help you open jars and bottles or to turn the door knobs in your house more easily.

In addition, there are also medicines that can help with the pain and swelling. Acetaminophen can safely ease arthritis pain. Some NSAIDs (**n**onsteroidal **a**nti-**i**nflammatory **d**rugs), like ibuprofen and naproxen, are sold without a prescription. Other NSAIDs must be prescribed by a doctor. But in 2005, the Food and Drug Administration (FDA) warned people about the possible side effects of some NSAIDs, both those sold with or without a prescription. You should read the warnings on the package or insert that comes with the drug. Talk to your doctor about if and how you should use acetaminophen or NSAIDs for your arthritis pain. You can also check with the FDA for more information about these drugs.

Some treatments are special for each common type of arthritis.

Osteoarthritis. Medicines can help you control OA pain. Rest and exercise will make it easier for you to move your joints. Keeping your weight down is a good idea. If pain from OA in your knee is very bad, your doctor might give you shots in the joint. This can help you to move your knee and get about without pain. Some people have surgery to repair or replace damaged joints.

Rheumatoid Arthritis. With treatment, the pain and swelling from RA will get better, and joint damage might slow down or stop. You may find it easier to move around, and you will just feel better. In addition to pain and anti-inflammatory medicines, your doctor might suggest antirheumatic drugs, called DMARDs (**d**isease-**m**odifying **a**nti**r**heumatic **d**rugs). These can slow damage from the disease. Medicines like prednisone, known as corticosteroids, can ease swelling while you wait for DMARDs to take effect. Another type of drug, biologic response modifiers, blocks the damage done by the immune system. They sometimes help people with mild-to-moderate RA when other treatments have not worked.

Gout. If you have had an attack of gout, talk to your doctor to learn why you had the attack and how to prevent future attacks. The most common treatment for an acute attack of gout uses NSAIDs or corticosteroids like prednisone. This reduces swelling, so you may start to feel better within a few hours after treatment. The attack usually goes away fully within a few days. If you have had several attacks, your doctor can prescribe medicines to prevent future ones.

Exercise Can Help

Along with taking the right medicine and properly resting your joints, exercise is a good way to stay fit, keep muscles strong, and control arthritis symptoms. Daily exercise, such as walking or swimming, helps keep joints moving, lessens pain, and makes muscles around the joints stronger.

Three types of exercise are best if you have arthritis:

- *Range-of-motion* exercises, like dancing, relieve stiffness, keep you flexible, and help you keep moving your joints.
- *Strengthening* exercises, such as weight training, will keep or add to muscle strength. Strong muscles support and protect your joints.
- *Aerobic or endurance* exercises, like bicycle riding, make your heart and arteries healthier, help prevent weight gain, and improve the overall working of your body. Aerobic exercise also may lessen swelling in some joints.

The National Institute on Aging (NIA) has a free 80-page booklet on how to start and stick with a safe exercise program. The Institute also has a 48-minute companion video. See the last page of this *Age Page* for more information. Before beginning any exercise program, talk with your doctor or health care worker.

Other Things to Do

Along with exercise and weight control, there are other ways to ease the pain around joints. You might find comfort by applying heat or cold, soaking in a warm bath, or swimming in a heated pool.

Your doctor may suggest surgery when damage to your joints becomes disabling or when other treatments do not help with pain. Surgeons can repair or replace these joints with artificial (man-made) ones. In the most common operations, doctors replace hips and knees.

Unproven Remedies

Many people with arthritis try remedies that have not been tested or proved to be helpful. Some of these, such as snake venom, are harmful. Others, such as copper bracelets, are harmless, but also unproven.

How can you tell that a remedy may be unproven?

- The remedy claims that a treatment, like a lotion or cream, works for all types of arthritis and other diseases,
- Scientific support comes from only one research study, or
- The label has no directions for use or warning about side effects.

Areas for Further Research

Recent studies suggest that Chinese acupuncture may ease OA pain for some people. Others try dietary supplements, such as glucosamine and chondroitin. Research now shows that these two dietary supplements may help lessen your OA pain. Scientists are studying alternative treatments, such as these two supplements,

ARTHRITIS ADVICE 7

to find out how they work and if they keep the joint changes caused by arthritis from getting worse. More information is needed before anyone can be sure.

Talk to Your Doctor

Most importantly, do not take for granted that your pain and arthritis are just part of growing older normally. You and your doctor can work together to safely lessen the pain and stiffness that might be troubling you and to prevent more serious damage to your joints.

For More Information

Here are other resources about arthritis:

National Center for Complementary and Alternative Medicine
NCCAM Clearinghouse
P.O. Box 7923
Gaithersburg, MD 20898
888-644-6226 (toll-free)
866-464-3615 (TTY/toll-free)
www.nccam.nih.gov

National Institute of Arthritis and Musculoskeletal and Skin Diseases
NIAMS Information Clearinghouse
1 AMS Circle
Bethesda, MD 20892–3675
301-495-4484
877-226-4267 (toll-free)
301-565–2966 (TTY)
www.niams.nih.gov

American College of Rheumatology/Association of Rheumatology Health Professionals
1800 Century Place, Suite 250
Atlanta, GA 30345-4300
404-633-3777
www.rheumatology.org

Arthritis Foundation
P.O. Box 7669
Atlanta, GA 30357-0669
800-283-7800 (toll-free)
www.arthritis.org

- Check the telephone directory for your local chapter.

To get the NIA's exercise book or video or for more information about health and aging, call or write:

National Institute on Aging Information Center
P.O. Box 8057
Gaithersburg, MD 20898-8057
800-222-2225 (toll-free)
800-222-4225 (TTY/toll-free)

- To order publications (in English or Spanish) online, visit www.niapublications.org.
- The National Institute on Aging website is www.nia.nih.gov.
- Visit NIHSeniorHealth.gov (www.nihseniorhealth.gov), a senior-friendly website from the National Institute on Aging and the National Library of Medicine. This simple-to-use website features popular health topics for older adults. It has large type and a "talking" function that reads the text out loud.

May 2005

Cancer Facts for People Over 50

Cancer strikes people of all ages, but you are more likely to get cancer as you get older, even if no one in your family has had it. The good news is that the chances of surviving cancer are better today than ever before.

When cancer is found early, it is more likely to be treated successfully. You can help safeguard your health by learning the warning signs of cancer and by having regular checkups.

What Symptoms Should I Watch for?

You should see your doctor for regular checkups; don't wait for problems to occur. But you also should know that the following symptoms may be signs of cancer:

- Changes in bowel or bladder habits,
- A sore that does not heal,
- Unusual bleeding or discharge,
- Thickening or lump in the breast or any other part of the body,
- Indigestion or difficulty swallowing,
- Obvious change in a wart or mole,
- Nagging cough or hoarseness, or
- Unexplained changes in weight.

What If I Have One of These Symptoms?

These symptoms are not always a sign of cancer. They also can be caused by less serious conditions. It's important to see a doctor if you have symptoms because only a doctor can make a diagnosis. **Don't** wait to feel pain! Early cancer usually doesn't cause pain.

Some people believe that as they age their symptoms are due to "growing older." Because of this myth, many illnesses go undiagnosed and untreated. Don't ignore your symptoms because you think they are not important or because you believe they are normal for your age. Talk to your doctor.

What Regular Tests Should I Have?

Most cancers in their earliest, most treatable stages don't cause any symptoms or pain. That is why it's important to have regular tests to check for cancer long before you might notice anything wrong.

Checking for cancer in a person who does not have any symptoms is called screening. Screening may involve a physical exam, lab tests, or procedures to look at internal organs. Medicare now covers a number of screening tests for cancer. For details, check with the Medicare toll-free help line at 800-633-4227.

Before recommending a screening test, your doctor will consider your age, medical history, general health, family history, and lifestyle. You may want to discuss your concerns or questions with your doctor, so that together you can weigh the pros and cons and make an informed decision about whether to have a screening test. If you are 50 or older, the following are some of the cancer screening tests that you and your doctor should consider:

- *Mammogram.* A woman's risk of breast cancer increases with age; about 80 percent of breast cancers occur in women over age 50. A mammogram is a special x-ray of the breast that often can find cancers that are too small for a woman or her doctor to feel. The National Cancer Institute (NCI) recommends that women in their 40s or older have a screening mammogram on a regular basis, every 1–2 years.

- *Clinical Breast Exam.* During a clinical breast exam, the doctor or other health care professional checks the breasts and underarms for lumps or other changes that could be a sign of breast cancer.

- *Fecal Occult Blood Test.* Colorectal cancer is the third leading cause of death from cancer in the United States. The risk of developing colorectal cancer rises after age 50. It is common in both men and women. Studies show that a fecal occult blood test every 1–2 years in people between the ages of 50 and 80 decreases the number of deaths due to colorectal cancer. For this test, stool samples are applied to special cards, which are examined in a lab for occult (hidden) blood.

- *Sigmoidoscopy.* A doctor uses a thin, flexible tube with a light (sigmoidoscope) to look inside the colon and rectum for growths or abnormal areas. Fewer people may die of colorectal cancer if they have regular screening by sigmoidoscopy after age 50.

- *Pap Test.* The risk of cancer of the cervix (the lower, narrow part of the uterus or womb) increases with age. Most invasive cancers of the cervix can be prevented if women have Pap tests and pelvic exams regularly. Older women should continue to have regular Pap tests and pelvic exams. The doctor uses a wooden scraper or a small brush to collect a sample of cells from the cervix and upper vagina. The cells are sent to a lab to check for abnormalities.

- *Pelvic Exam.* In a pelvic exam, the doctor checks the uterus, vagina, ovaries, fallopian tubes, bladder, and rectum for any changes in their shape or size. During a pelvic exam, an instrument called a speculum is used to widen the vagina so that the upper part of the vagina and the cervix can be seen.

- *Digital Rectal Exam.* Prostate cancer is the most common cancer in American men—especially older men. More than 80 percent of prostate cancers occur in men 65 and older. Research is being done to find the most reliable screening test for prostate cancer. Scientists at the NCI are studying the value of digital rectal exam and prostate-specific antigen (PSA) in reducing the number of deaths caused by prostate cancer. For a digital rectal exam, the doctor inserts a gloved finger into the rectum and feels the prostate gland for bumps or abnormal areas.

- *Prostate Specific Antigen (PSA).* This test measures the amount of PSA in the blood-stream. Higher-than-average amounts of PSA may indicate the presence of prostate cancer cells. However, PSA levels also may be high in men who have noncancerous prostate conditions. Scientists are studying ways to improve the validity of the PSA test.

- *Skin Exam.* Skin cancer is the most common form of cancer in the United States. Routine examination of the skin increases the chance of finding skin cancer early.

A positive result on any of these tests doesn't mean that you have cancer. You may need more tests. A biopsy is the only sure way to know whether the problem is cancer. In this test, a sample of tissue is removed from the abnormal area and examined under a microscope to check for cancer cells.

What if I'm Told I Have Cancer?

If tests show that you have cancer, you should talk with your doctor and make treatment decisions as soon as possible. Cancer is a disease in which cells become abnormal and keep dividing and forming more cells without order or control. If left untreated, cancer cells can damage nearby tissues and organs. Cancer cells also can break away and spread to other parts of the body. Thus, early treatment means better outcomes.

How is Cancer Treated?

There are a number of cancer treatments, including surgery, radiation therapy, chemotherapy (anticancer drugs), and biological therapy (treatment that uses the body's natural ability to fight infection and disease). Patients with cancer often are treated by a team of specialists, which may include a medical oncologist (specialist in cancer treatment), a surgeon, a radiation oncologist (specialist in radiation therapy), and others. The doctors may decide to use one type of treatment alone or a combination of treatments. The choice of treatment depends on the type and location of the cancer, the stage of the disease, the patient's general health, and other factors.

Before starting treatment, you may want another doctor to review the diagnosis and treatment plan. Some insurance companies require a second opinion; others may pay for a second opinion if you request it.

Some cancer patients take part in studies of new treatments. These studies—called clinical trials—are designed to find out whether a new treatment is both safe and effective. Often, clinical trials compare a new treatment with a standard one so that doctors can learn which is more effective. Clinical trials offer important choices for many patients. Cancer patients who are interested in taking part in a clinical trial should talk with their doctor.

Can Cancer be Prevented?

Although your chances of getting cancer increase after age 50, there are things that you can do to prevent it. About 80 percent of all cancers are related to the use of tobacco products, to what we eat and drink, or to a lesser extent to exposure to radiation or cancer-causing agents in the environment and the workplace. Many risk factors can be avoided:

- Do not use tobacco products. Tobacco causes cancer. In fact, smoking tobacco, using smokeless tobacco, and being exposed regularly to involuntary tobacco smoke are responsible for one-third of all cancer deaths in the United States each year.

- Avoid the harmful rays of the sun. Ultraviolet radiation from the sun and from other sources—such as sunlamps and tanning booths—damages your skin and can cause skin cancer.

- Choose foods with less fat and more fiber. Your choice of foods may affect your chance of developing cancer. Evidence points to a link between a high-fat diet and cancers of the breast, colon, uterus, and prostate. Being seriously overweight appears to be linked to cancers of the prostate, pancreas, uterus, colon, and ovary and to breast cancer in older women. On the other hand, you may be able to reduce your cancer risk by making some simple food choices. Try to eat a varied, well-balanced diet that includes generous amounts of foods that are high in fiber, vitamins, and minerals. Aim for at least five servings of fruits and vegetables each day. At the same time, try to cut down on fatty foods.

- If you drink alcohol, do so in moderation—not more than one or two drinks a day. Drinking large amounts of alcohol increases the risk of cancers of the mouth, throat, esophagus, and larynx. People who smoke cigarettes and drink alcohol have an especially high risk of getting these cancers.

For More Information

The organizations listed below offer more information about some of the topics mentioned in this fact sheet:

The Cancer Information Service (CIS), a program of the National Cancer Institute, can provide accurate, up-to-date information about cancer. Information specialists can answer your questions in English, Spanish, and on TTY equipment.
800-422-6237 (toll-free)
800-332-8615 (TTY/toll-free)

For more information about health and aging, contact:

National Institute on Aging Information Center
P.O. Box 8057
Gaithersburg, MD 20898-8057
800-222-2225 (toll-free)
800-222-4225 (TTY/toll-free)

- To order publications (in English or Spanish) online, visit www.niapublications.org.

- The National Institute on Aging website is www.nia.nih.gov.

- Visit NIHSeniorHealth.gov (*www.nihseniorhealth.gov*), a senior-friendly website from the National Institute on Aging and the National Library of Medicine. This simple-to-use website features popular health topics for older adults. It has large type and a "talking" function that reads the text out loud.

2000

Depression: Don't Let the Blues Hang Around

Everyone feels blue now and then. It's part of life. But if you no longer enjoy activities that you usually like, you may have a more serious problem. Being depressed, without letup, can change the way you think and feel. Doctors call this medical disorder "clinical depression."

Being "down in the dumps" over a period of time is not a normal part of getting older. But it is a common problem, and medical help may be needed. For most people, depression will get better with treatment. "Talk" therapy, medicine, or other treatment methods can ease the pain of depression. You do not need to suffer.

There are many reasons why depression in older people is often hard to detect and treat. As a person ages, the signs of depression are much more varied than at younger ages. It can appear as increased tiredness, or it can be seen as grumpiness. Sometimes people who are depressed lose interest in eating and can lose weight. Confusion or attention problems caused by depression can sometimes look like Alzheimer's disease or other brain disorders. Mood changes and signs of depression can be caused by medicines older people may take for arthritis, high blood pressure, or heart disease. The good news is that people who are depressed usually feel better with the right treatment.

What Causes Depression?

There is no one cause of depression. For some people, a single event can bring on the illness. Depression often strikes people who suddenly have to deal with a serious illness or a death in the family. For some people, a loss in their own physical or mental skills brings on depression. Sometimes those under a lot of stress, like caregivers, can feel depressed. Others become depressed for no clear reason.

People with serious illnesses, such as cancer, diabetes, heart disease, stroke, or Parkinson's disease, sometimes become depressed. They worry about how their illness will change their lives. They might be tired and not able to deal with something that makes them sad. Treatment for depression helps them feel better and improves quality of life.

Genetics, too, can play a role. Studies show that depression may run in families. Children of depressed parents may be at a higher risk for depression. And, depression tends to be a disorder that occurs more than once. Many older people who have been depressed in the past are at an increased risk.

What to Look For

How do you know when you need help? After all, as you age, you may have to face problems that could cause anyone to feel "depressed." Perhaps you are dealing with the death of a loved one or friend. Maybe you are having a tough time getting used to retirement, and you feel lonely. Possibly you have a chronic illness. Or, you might feel like you have lost control over your life.

After a period of feeling sad, older people usually adjust and regain their emotional balance. But, if you are suffering from clinical depression and don't get help, your depression might last for weeks, months, or even years. Here is a list of the most common signs of depression. If you have several of these, and they last for more than 2 weeks, see a doctor.

- An "empty" feeling, ongoing sadness, and anxiety,
- Tiredness, lack of energy,
- Loss of interest or pleasure in everyday activities, including sex,
- Sleep problems, including trouble getting to sleep, very early morning waking, and sleeping too much,
- Eating more or less than usual,
- Crying too often or too much,
- Aches and pains that don't go away when treated,
- A hard time focusing, remembering, or making decisions,
- Feeling guilty, helpless, worthless, or hopeless,
- Being irritable, or
- Thoughts of death or suicide; a suicide attempt.

If you are a family member, friend, or health care provider of an older person, watch carefully for clues of depression. Sometimes symptoms can hide behind a smiling face. A depressed person who lives alone may appear to feel better when someone stops by to say hello. The symptoms may seem to go away. But, when someone is very depressed, the symptoms usually come back.

Don't ignore the warning signs. If left untreated, serious depression can lead to suicide. Listen carefully if someone of any age complains about being depressed or says people don't care. That person may really be asking for help.

Getting Help

The first step is to accept that you or your family member needs help. You may not be comfortable with the subject of depression and mental illness. Or, you might feel that asking for help is a sign of weakness. You might be like many older people, their relatives, or friends, who believe that a depressed person can quickly "snap out of it" or that some people are too old to be helped. This is wrong.

A health care provider can help. Once you decide to get medical advice, start with your family doctor. The doctor should check to see if your depression could be caused by a health problem (such as hypothyroidism or vitamin B_{12} deficiency) or a medicine you are taking. After a complete exam, your doctor may suggest you talk to a mental health worker, such as a social worker, mental health counselor, psychologist, or psychiatrist. Doctors specially trained to treat depression in older people are called geriatric psychiatrists.

Don't avoid getting help because you may be afraid of how much treatment might cost. Often, only short-term psychotherapy (talk therapy) is needed. It is usually covered by insurance. Also, some community mental health centers may offer treatment based on a person's ability to pay.

Be aware that some family doctors may not understand about aging and depression. If your doctor is unable or unwilling to help, you may want to talk to another health care provider.

Are you the relative or friend of a depressed older person who won't go to a doctor for treatment? Try explaining how treatment may help the person feel better. In some cases, when a depressed person can't or won't go to the doctor's office, the doctor or mental health expert can start by making a phone call. A telephone call can't take the place of the personal contact needed for a complete medical checkup, but it might encourage the person to go for treatment.

Treating Depression

Your doctor or mental health expert can often treat your depression successfully. Different therapies seem to work for different people. For instance, support groups can provide new coping skills or social support if you are dealing with a major life change. A doctor might suggest that you go to a local senior center, volunteer service, or nutrition program.

Several kinds of talk therapies are useful as well. One method might help give you a more positive outlook on life. Always thinking about the sad things in your life or what you have lost might have led to your depression. Another method works to improve your relations with others to give you more hope about the future.

Getting better takes time, but with support from others and treatment you will get a little better each day.

Antidepressant drugs (medicine to treat depression) can also help. These medications can improve your mood, sleep, appetite, and concentration. There are several types of antidepressants available. Some of these medicines must be taken for as long as 12 weeks before you feel like they are working. Your doctor may want you to continue medications for 6 months or more after your symptoms disappear.

Some antidepressants can cause unwanted side effects, although newer medicines have fewer side effects. Any antidepressant should be used with great care to avoid this problem. Remember:

- The doctor needs to know about all prescribed and over-the-counter medications, vitamins, or herbal supplements you are taking.
- The doctor should also be aware of any other physical problems you have.
- Be sure to take antidepressants in the proper dose and on the right schedule.

Electroconvulsive therapy (ECT) can also help. Don't be misled by the way some movies and books have portrayed ECT (also called electroshock therapy). They do not give a true picture. ECT may be recommended when medicines can't be tolerated or when a quick response is needed. ECT is given as a series of treatments over a few weeks and is very safe and effective. Like other antidepressant therapies, follow-up treatment is often needed to help prevent a return of depression.

Help from Family and Friends

Family and friends can play an important role in treatment. You can help your relative or friend stay with the treatment plan. If needed, make appointments for the person or go along to the doctor, mental health expert, or support group.

Be patient and understanding. Get your relative or friend to go on outings with you or to go back to an activity that he or she once enjoyed. Encourage the person to be active and busy, but not to take on too much at one time.

Preventing Depression

What can be done to lower the risk of depression? How can people cope? There are a few steps you can take. Try to prepare for major changes in life, such as retirement or moving from your home of many years. One way to do this is to try and keep friendships over the years. Friends can help ease loneliness if you lose a spouse. You can also develop a hobby. Hobbies may help keep your mind and body active. Stay in touch with family. Let them help you when you feel very sad. If you are faced with a lot to do, try to break it up into smaller jobs that are easier to finish.

Exercise can help prevent depression or lift your mood if you are already depressed. Older people who are depressed can gain mental as well as physical benefits from mild forms of exercise like walking outdoors or in shopping malls. Gardening, dancing, and swimming are other good forms of exercise. Pick something you like to do. Begin with 10-15 minutes a day, and increase the time as you are able. Being physically fit and eating a balanced diet may help avoid illnesses that can bring on disability or depression.

Remember, with treatment, most people will find positive thoughts gradually replacing negative thoughts. Expect your mood to improve slowly. Feeling better takes time. But it can happen.

For More Information

The following groups offer information on depression and older people:

American Association for Geriatric Psychiatry (AAGP)
7910 Woodmont Avenue
Suite 1050
Bethesda, MD 20814-3004
301-654-7850
www.aagpgpa.org

American Psychological Association (APA)
750 First Street, NE
Washington, DC 20002
800-374-2721 (toll-free)
www.apa.org

Depression and Bipolar Support Alliance (DBSA)
730 North Franklin Street
Suite 501
Chicago, IL 60610-7204
800-826-3632 (toll-free)
www.dbsalliance.org

National Alliance for the Mentally Ill
Colonial Place Three
2107 Wilson Boulevard
Suite 300
Arlington, VA 22201
800-950-6264 (toll-free)
www.nami.org

National Institute of Mental Health (NIMH)
6001 Executive Boulevard
Room 8184, MSC 9663
Bethesda, MD 20892-9663
301-443-4513
301-443-8431 (TTY)
www.nimh.nih.gov

- For publications, call 800-421-4211 (toll-free)

National Mental Health Association (NMHA)
2001 North Beauregard Street
12th Floor
Alexandria, VA 22311
800-969-6642 (toll-free)
800-433-5959 (TTY/toll-free)
www.nmha.org

For information about depression and Alzheimer's patients and caregivers, contact:

Alzheimer's Disease Education and Referral (ADEAR) Center
P.O. Box 8250
Silver Spring, MD 20907-8250
800-438-4380 (toll-free)
www.alzheimers.org

For more information about health and aging, contact

National Institute on Aging Information Center
P.O. Box 8057
Gaithersburg, MD 20898-8057
800-222-2225 (toll-free)
800-222-4225 (TTY/toll-free)

- To order publications (in English or Spanish) online, visit www.niapublications.org.
- The National Institute on Aging website is www.nia.nih.gov.
- Visit NIHSeniorHealth.gov (www.nihseniorhealth.gov), a senior-friendly website from the National Institute on Aging and the National Library of Medicine. This simple-to-use website features popular health topics for older adults. It has large type and a "talking" function that reads the text out loud.

April 2005

Diabetes in Older People — A Disease You Can Manage

Diabetes is a serious disease. It happens when your blood levels of glucose, a form of sugar, are too high. Diabetes can lead to dangerous health problems. The good news is that high glucose levels can be managed to help control the disease and prevent or delay future problems.

What is Diabetes?

Our bodies change the foods we eat into glucose. Glucose travels through the bloodstream to "fuel" or feed our cells. Insulin is a hormone that helps our bodies use glucose for energy. People with diabetes either do not make insulin, do not use insulin properly, or both. This means they have too much glucose (sugar) in their blood. As a result, they often feel tired, hungry, or thirsty; they may lose weight, urinate often, or have trouble with their eyes. In time, the high levels of this form of sugar in the blood (glucose) can hurt their eyes, kidneys, and nerves. It can also cause heart disease, strokes, and even the need to remove all or part of a limb (amputation).

Diabetes tends to run in families, but other factors add to the risk of getting diabetes. For example, being overweight and underactive can sometimes trigger diabetes in people who are at risk. There is a lot of research underway looking at what causes diabetes and how best to manage it.

But there is a lot we do know. For example, we know that careful control of blood glucose, blood pressure, and cholesterol can help prevent or delay diabetes and its complications.

Types of Diabetes

There are two types of diabetes. In one kind, people must take insulin every day. This is called *type 1 diabetes*, formerly known as *juvenile-onset diabetes*. Type 1 diabetes is often first seen in children, teenagers, or adults under age 30.

The second kind of diabetes happens when the body produces insulin but doesn't *use* it in the right way. This is called *type 2 diabetes*, formerly called *adult-onset diabetes*. It is most common in people over age 40. Type 2 diabetes is linked to obesity, lack of activity, family history of diabetes, and family background. African Americans, Hispanic/Latino Americans, American Indians, and some Asian Americans and Pacific Islanders are at very high risk for type 2 diabetes.

There is also a condition called *pre-diabetes* in which blood glucose (a form of sugar) levels are higher than normal but not high enough to be called diabetes. This condition raises the risk of type 2 diabetes, heart disease, and stroke.

People with pre-diabetes can delay or prevent type 2 diabetes by losing weight and being more active.

Related Health Concerns

Blood glucose levels that are either very high or very low can lead to serious medical problems, even emergencies. In addition to the health problems noted above, people with diabetes could go into a coma (become unconscious) if their blood glucose levels get very high. Low blood glucose (called hypoglycemia) can also cause problems if it's untreated. Usually hypoglycemia is mild and can easily be treated by eating or drinking something with carbohydrates such as bread, fruit, potatoes, or milk. But, left untreated, hypoglycemia can lead to loss of consciousness. Although hypoglycemia can happen suddenly, it can usually be treated quickly, bringing your blood glucose level back to normal.

Researchers recently have found that people with diabetes also have an increased risk for Alzheimer's disease. Studies are underway to understand this connection and to see whether strict control of glucose can delay or prevent this problem.

Symptoms

Often, people with type 2 diabetes have few or no symptoms. Many people with type 2 diabetes don't even know they have it. For some people, feeling rundown is their only symptom. Other people may feel thirsty, urinate often, lose weight, have blurred vision, get skin infections, or heal slowly from cuts and bruises. It is very important to tell the doctor right away about *any* of these problems.

Tests

Medical tests will show if diabetes is causing your problems. A doctor can diagnose diabetes by reviewing your symptoms and checking your blood glucose levels. One test (*fasting plasma glucose test*) measures your blood glucose level after eating or drinking nothing (fasting) for at least eight hours, usually overnight. In another test, called the *oral glucose tolerance test*, your blood glucose is checked and then you drink a sugary beverage. Your blood glucose (sugar) levels are then checked 1 hour, 2 hours, and 3 hours later. Diagnosis is confirmed after a repeat test on a different day.

Research shows that some increase in blood glucose levels often comes with age. This may be caused by weight gain, especially when fat builds up around the waist.

Managing Diabetes

There are things you can do to take control of your diabetes.

- Meal planning and eating correctly are key to managing blood glucose, blood pressure, and cholesterol levels. To plan meals and eat right, you need to understand how different foods affect your glucose levels. A good meal plan will take into account your food likes and dislikes, goals for weight control, and daily physical activity. Health care professionals can work with you to create a personalized meal plan.

- Physical activity is very important in dealing with diabetes. Taking part in a regular fitness program can improve blood glucose levels in older people with diabetes. A health care professional can help plan a physical activity program just right for you.

- Medications are also central to controlling diabetes for many people. Doctors may prescribe oral medicines (those taken by mouth), insulin, or a combination of both as needed. People with type 2 diabetes may not need to take diabetes medications if they can reach glucose, blood pressure, and cholesterol goals through meal planning, eating the right foods, and physical activity.

- Keeping track of how well your diabetes care plan is working is important. Check blood glucose levels and monitor your blood pressure and cholesterol levels.

What Else Can You Do?

Eye Exams. People with diabetes should have an eye exam every year. Finding and treating eye problems early can help prevent more serious conditions later on.

Kidney Check. A yearly urine test for a protein called albumin will show whether your kidneys are affected by diabetes.

Foot Care. Diabetes can reduce blood supply to arms and legs and cause numbness in the feet. People with diabetes should check their feet every day and watch for any redness or patches of heat. Sores, blisters, breaks in the skin, infections, or build-up of calluses should be checked right away by a doctor specializing in foot care (podiatrist) or a family doctor.

Skin Care. People with diabetes can protect their skin by keeping it clean, using skin softeners to treat dryness, and taking care of minor cuts and bruises to prevent infections and other problems.

Care of Teeth and Gums. Working closely with a dentist is very important. Teeth and gums need special attention to avoid serious infections.

Flu Shots and Pneumonia Vaccine. Getting a yearly flu shot and a pneumonia vaccine at least once will help keep people with diabetes healthy. If five years or more have passed since your pneumonia shot, ask your doctor if you should be revaccinated.

People with diabetes who are on Medicare now receive coverage for supplies such as glucose monitors, test strips, and lancets. For more information about what is covered, call 800-MEDICARE (800-633-4227).

For More Information

The following organizations offer a wealth of information, as well as free or low-cost resources for people with diabetes, health care professionals, and the general public:

National Diabetes Education Program
One Diabetes Way
Bethesda, MD 20814-9692
800-438-5383 (toll-free)
www.ndep.nih.gov

American Diabetes Association
1701 North Beauregard Street
Alexandria, VA 22311
800-342-2383 (toll-free)
www.diabetes.org

National Institute of Diabetes and Digestive and Kidney Diseases
National Diabetes Information Clearinghouse
One Information Way
Bethesda, MD 20892-3560
800-860-8747 (toll-free)
301-654-4415
www.diabetes.niddk.nih.gov

For more information about health and aging, contact:

National Institute on Aging Information Center
P.O. Box 8057
Gaithersburg, MD 20898-8057
800-222-2225 (toll-free)
800-222-4225 (TTY/toll-free)

- To order publications (in English or Spanish) online, visit *www.niapublications.org.*

- The National Institute on Aging website is *www.nia.nih.gov.*

- Visit NIHSeniorHealth.gov (*www.nihseniorhealth.gov*), a senior-friendly website from the National Institute on Aging and the National Library of Medicine. This simple-to-use website features popular health topics for older adults. It has large type and a "talking" function that reads the text out loud.

July 2004

Forgetfulness: It's Not Always What You Think

Many older people worry about becoming more forgetful. They think forgetfulness is the first sign of Alzheimer's disease. In the past, memory loss and confusion were considered a normal part of aging. However, scientists now know that most people remain both alert and able as they age, although it may take them longer to remember things.

A lot of people experience memory lapses. Some memory problems are serious, and others are not. People who have serious changes in their memory, personality, and behavior may suffer from a form of brain disease called dementia. Dementia seriously affects a person's ability to carry out daily activities. Alzheimer's disease is one of many types of dementia.

The term dementia describes a group of symptoms that are caused by changes in brain function. Dementia symptoms may include asking the same questions repeatedly; becoming lost in familiar places; being unable to follow directions; getting disoriented about time, people, and places; and neglecting personal safety, hygiene, and nutrition. People with dementia lose their abilities at different rates. Dementia is caused by many conditions. Some conditions that cause dementia can be reversed, and others cannot. Further, many different medical conditions may cause symptoms that seem like Alzheimer's disease, but are not. Some of these medical conditions may be treatable. Reversible conditions can be caused by a high fever, dehydration, vitamin deficiency and poor nutrition, bad reactions to medicines, problems with the thyroid gland, or a minor head injury. Medical conditions like these can be serious and should be treated by a doctor as soon as possible.

Sometimes older people have emotional problems that can be mistaken for dementia. Feeling sad, lonely, worried, or bored may be more common for older people facing retirement or coping with the death of a spouse, relative, or friend. Adapting to these changes leaves some people feeling confused or forgetful. Emotional problems can be eased by supportive friends and family or by professional help from a doctor or counselor.

The two most common forms of dementia in older people are Alzheimer's disease and multi-infarct dementia (sometimes called vascular dementia). These types of dementia are irreversible, which means they cannot be cured. In Alzheimer's disease, nerve cell changes in certain parts of the brain result in the death of a large number of cells. Symptoms of Alzheimer's disease begin slowly and become steadily worse. As the disease progresses, symptoms range from mild forgetfulness to serious impairments in thinking, judgment, and the ability to perform daily activities. Eventually, patients may need total care.

In multi-infarct dementia, a series of small strokes or changes in the brain's blood supply may result in the death of brain tissue. The location in the brain where the small strokes occur determines the seriousness of the problem and the symptoms that arise. Symptoms that begin suddenly may be a sign of this kind of dementia. People with multi-infarct dementia are likely to show signs of improvement or remain stable for long periods of time, then quickly develop new symptoms if more strokes occur. In many people with multi-infarct dementia, high blood pressure is to blame. One of the most important reasons for controlling high blood pressure is to prevent strokes.

Diagnosis

People who are worried about memory problems should see their doctor. If the doctor believes that the problem is serious, then a thorough physical, neurological, and psychiatric evaluation may be recommended. A complete medical examination for memory loss may include gathering information about the person's medical history, including use of prescription and over-the-counter medicines, diet, past medical problems, and general health. Because a correct diagnosis depends on recalling these details accurately, the doctor also may ask a family member for information about the person.

Tests of blood and urine may be done to help the doctor find any problems. There are also tests of mental abilities (tests of memory, problem solving, counting, and language). A brain CT scan may assist the doctor in ruling out a curable disorder. A scan also may show signs of normal age-related changes in the brain. It may be necessary to have another scan at a later date to see if there have been further changes in the brain.

Alzheimer's disease and multi-infarct dementia can exist together, making it hard for the doctor to diagnose either one specifically. Scientists once thought that multi-infarct dementia and other types of vascular dementia caused most cases of irreversible mental impairment. They now believe that most older people with irreversible dementia have Alzheimer's disease.

Treatment

Even if the doctor diagnoses an irreversible form of dementia, much still can be done to treat the patient and help the family cope. A person with dementia should be under a doctor's care and may see a neurologist, psychiatrist, family doctor, internist, or geriatrician. The doctor can treat the patient's physical and behavioral problems and answer the many questions that the person or family may have.

For some people in the early and middle stages of Alzheimer's disease, the drugs tacrine (Cognex), donepezil (Aricept), rivastigmine (Exelon), and galantamine (Reminyl) are prescribed to possibly delay the worsening of some of the disease's symptoms. Another drug, memantine (Namenda), has been approved for treatment of moderate to severe AD. Doctors believe it is very important for people with multi-infarct dementia to try to prevent further strokes by controlling high blood pressure, monitoring and treating high blood cholesterol and diabetes, and not smoking.

Many people with dementia need no medication for behavioral problems. But for some people, doctors may prescribe medications to reduce agitation, anxiety, depression, or sleeping problems. These troublesome behaviors are common in people with dementia. Careful use of doctor-prescribed drugs may make some people with dementia more comfortable and make caring for them easier.

A healthy diet is important. Although no special diets or nutritional supplements have been found to prevent or reverse Alzheimer's disease or multi-infarct dementia, a balanced diet helps maintain overall good health. In cases of multi-infarct dementia, improving the diet may play a role in preventing more strokes.

Family members and friends can assist people with dementia in continuing their daily routines, physical activities, and social contacts. People with dementia should be kept up-to-date about the details of their lives, such as the time of day, where they live, and what is happening at home or in the world. Memory aids may help in the day-to-day living of patients in the earlier stages of dementia. Some families find that a big calendar, a list of daily plans, notes about simple safety measures, and written directions describing how to use common household items are very useful aids.

Advice for Today

Scientists are working to develop new drugs that someday may slow, reverse, or prevent the damage caused by Alzheimer's disease and multi-infarct dementia. In the meantime, people who have no dementia symptoms can try to keep their memory sharp.

Some suggestions include developing interests or hobbies and staying involved in activities that stimulate both the mind and body. Giving careful attention to physical fitness and exercise also may go a long way toward keeping a healthy state of mind. Limiting the use of alcoholic beverages is important, because heavy drinking over time can cause permanent brain damage.

Many people find it useful to plan tasks, make "things to do" lists, and use notes, calendars, and other memory aids. They also may remember things better by mentally connecting them to other meaningful things, such as a familiar name, song, or lines from a poem.

Stress, anxiety, or depression can make a person more forgetful. Forgetfulness caused by these emotions usually is temporary and goes away when the feelings fade. However, if these feelings last for a long period of time, getting help from a professional is important. Treatment may include counseling or medication, or a combination of both.

Some physical and mental changes occur with age in healthy people. However, much pain and suffering can be avoided if older people, their families, and their doctors recognize dementia as a disease, not part of normal aging.

For More Information

The organizations listed below offer more information about some of the topics mentioned in this fact sheet:

Alzheimer's Association
225 North Michigan Avenue
Suite 1700
Chicago, IL 60601-7633
800-272-3900 (toll-free)
e-mail: info@alz.org
www.alz.org

- The Alzheimer's Association is a nonprofit organization supporting AD research and offering information and support services to people with AD and their families.

ADEAR Center
P.O. Box 8250
Silver Spring, MD 20907-8250
800-438-4380 (toll-free)
e-mail: adear@alzheimers.org
www.alzheimers.org

- The Alzheimer's Disease Education and Referral (ADEAR) Center is a service of the National Institute on Aging, part of the Federal Government's National Institutes of Health. The Center provides information to health professionals, patients and their families, and the public. Information about community resources is available from State and Area Agencies on Aging.

Eldercare Locator
800-677-1116 (toll-free)
www.eldercare.gov

For more information about health and aging, contact:

National Institute on Aging Information Center
P.O. Box 8057
Gaithersburg, MD 20898-8057
800-222-2225 (toll-free)
800-222-4225 (TTY/toll-free)

- To order publications (in English or Spanish) online, visit www.niapublications.org.
- The National Institute on Aging website is www.nia.nih.gov.
- Visit NIHSeniorHealth.gov (www.nihseniorhealth.gov), a senior-friendly website from the National Institute on Aging and the National Library of Medicine. This simple-to-use website features popular health topics for older adults. It has large type and a "talking" function that reads the text out loud.

July 2004

Hearing Loss

About one-third of Americans older than age 60 have hearing problems. About half the people who are 85 and older have hearing loss. Whether a hearing loss is small (missing certain sounds) or large (being profoundly deaf), it is a serious concern. If left untreated, problems can get worse.

Hearing loss can affect your life in many ways. You may miss out on talks with friends and family. On the telephone, you may find it hard to hear what the caller is saying. At the doctor's office, you may not catch the doctor's words.

Sometimes hearing problems can make you feel embarrassed, upset, and lonely. It's easy to withdraw when you can't follow a conversation at the dinner table or in a restaurant. It's also easy for friends and family to think you are confused, uncaring, or difficult, when the problem may be that you just can't hear well.

If you have trouble hearing, there is help. Start by seeing your doctor. Depending on the type and extent of your hearing loss, there are many treatment choices that may help. Hearing loss does not have to get in the way of your ability to enjoy life.

How Do I Know if I Have a Hearing Loss?

See your doctor if you:

- Have trouble hearing over the telephone,
- Find it hard to follow conversations when two or more people are talking,
- Need to turn up the TV volume so loud that others complain,
- Have a problem hearing because of background noise,
- Sense that others seem to mumble, or
- Can't understand when women and children speak to you.

What Should I Do?

If you have trouble hearing, see your doctor. Sometimes the diagnosis and treatment can take place in the doctor's office. Or your doctor may refer you to an *otolaryngologist* (oh-toh-layr-ehn-GOL-luh-jist), a doctor who specializes in the ear, nose, and throat. The otolaryngologist will take a medical history, ask if other family members have hearing problems, do a thorough exam, and suggest any needed tests. You may be referred to an *audiologist* (aw-dee-AH-luh-jist). Audiologists are health care professionals trained to measure hearing. The audiologist will use an audiometer to test your ability to hear sounds of different pitch and loudness. These tests are painless. Audiologists can help if you need a hearing aid. They can help select the best hearing aid for you and help you learn to get the most from it.

What Causes Hearing Loss?

Hearing loss can have many different causes, including the aging process, ear wax buildup, exposure to very loud noises over a long period of time, viral or bacterial infections, heart conditions or stroke, head injuries, tumors, certain medicines, and heredity.

What Different Types of Hearing Loss Are There?

Presbycusis (prez-bee-KYOO-sis) is age-related hearing loss. It is common in people over the age of 50. People with this kind of hearing loss may have a hard time hearing what others are saying or may be unable to stand loud sounds. The decline is slow. Just as hair turns gray at different rates, presbycusis can develop at different rates. It can be caused by *sensorineural* (sen-soh-ree-NOO-ruhl) hearing loss. This type of hearing loss results from damage to parts of the inner ear, the auditory nerve, or hearing pathways in the brain. Presbycusis may be caused by aging, loud noise, heredity, head injury, infection, illness, certain prescription drugs, and circulation problems such as high blood pressure. The degree of hearing loss varies from person to person. Also, a person can have a different amount of hearing loss in each ear.

Tinnitus (tih-NIE-tuhs) accompanies many forms of hearing loss, including those that sometimes come with aging. People with tinnitus may hear a ringing, roaring, or some other noise inside their ears. Tinnitus may be caused by loud noise, hearing loss, certain medicines, and other health problems, such as allergies and problems in the heart and blood vessels. Often it is unclear why the ringing happens. Tinnitus can come and go, it can stop completely, or it can stay. Some medicines may help ease the problem. Wearing a hearing aid makes it easier for some people to hear the sounds they need to hear by making them louder. Maskers, small devices that use sound to make tinnitus less noticeable, help other people. Music also can be soothing and can sometimes mask the sounds caused by the condition. It also helps to avoid things that might make tinnitus worse, like smoking, alcohol, and loud noises.

Conductive hearing loss happens when something blocks the sounds that are carried from the eardrum (tympanic membrane) to the inner ear. Ear wax buildup, fluid in the middle ear, abnormal bone growth, a punctured eardrum, or a middle ear infection can cause this type of hearing loss. If ear wax blockage is a problem for you, the American Academy of Otolaryngology-Head and Neck Surgery suggests using mild treatments, such as mineral oil, baby oil, glycerin, or commercial ear drops to soften ear wax. If you think you may have a hole in your eardrum, however, you should see your doctor.

How Can I Help a Person with Hearing Loss?

Here are some tips you can use when talking with someone who has a hearing problem:

- Face the person, and talk clearly.
- Speak at a reasonable speed; do not hide your mouth, eat, or chew gum.

- Stand in good lighting, and reduce background noises.
- Use facial expressions or gestures to give useful clues.
- Repeat yourself if necessary, using different words.
- Include the hearing-impaired person when talking. Talk with the person, not about the person, when you are with others. This helps keep the hearing-impaired person from feeling alone and excluded.
- Be patient; stay positive and relaxed.
- Ask how you can help.

What Can I Do if I Have Trouble Hearing?

- Let people know that you have trouble hearing.
- Ask people to face you and to speak more slowly and clearly; also ask them to speak without shouting.
- Pay attention to what is being said and to facial expressions or gestures.
- Let the person talking know if you do not understand.
- Ask people to reword a sentence and try again.

What Devices or Treatments Can Help?

What will help you depends on your hearing problem. Some common solutions include:

Hearing aids. These are small devices you wear in or behind your ear. Hearing aids can help some kinds of hearing loss by making sounds louder. However, they sometimes pick up background noises—for example, traffic noise in the street or people talking at other tables in a crowded restaurant. This can affect how well you hear in certain situations. Before buying a hearing aid, check to find out if your insurance will cover the cost.

There are many kinds of hearing aids. An audiologist can help fit you with the hearing aid that will work best for you. You can ask the audiologist about having a trial period to try out a few different aids.

Remember, when you buy a hearing aid, you are buying a product and a service. Find a hearing aid dealer (called a dispenser) who has the patience and skill to help you during the month or so it takes to get used to the new hearing aid.

You may need to have several fittings of your hearing aid, and you will need to get directions on how to use it. Hearing aids use batteries, which you will need to change on a regular basis. They also may need repairs from time to time. Buy a hearing aid that has only the features you need.

Assistive/Adaptive Devices. There are many products that can help you live well with less-than-perfect hearing. The list below includes some examples of the many choices:

- *Telephone amplifying devices* range from a special type of telephone receiver that makes sounds louder to special phones that work with hearing aids.
- *TV and radio listening systems* can be used with or without hearing aids. You do not have to turn the volume up high.

- *Assistive listening devices* are available in some public places such as auditoriums, movie theaters, churches, synagogues, and meeting places.
- *Alerts* such as doorbells, smoke detectors, and alarm clocks can give you a signal that you can see or a vibration that you can feel. For example, a flashing light could let you know someone is at the door or that the phone is ringing.

Cochlear implants. If your deafness is severe, a doctor may suggest cochlear implants. In this surgery, the doctor puts a small electronic device under the skin behind the ear. The device sends the message past the non-working part of the inner ear and on to the brain. This process helps some people hear. These implants are not helpful for all types of deafness or hearing loss.

For More Information

There are many things you can do about hearing loss. The first step is to check with your doctor. You also can get more information from the following groups:

National Institute on Deafness and Other Communication Disorders (NIDCD)
NIDCD Information Clearinghouse
National Institutes of Health
31 Center Drive, MSC 2320
Bethesda, MD 20892-2320
800-241-1044 (toll-free)
800-241-1055 (TTY/toll-free)
www.nidcd.nih.gov

American Academy of Otolaryngology-Head and Neck Surgery, Inc. (AAO-HNS)
1 Prince Street
Alexandria, VA 22314-3357
703-836-4444
703-519-1585 (TTY)
www.entnet.org

American Speech-Language-Hearing Association (ASHA)
10801 Rockville Pike
Rockville, MD 20852
800-638-8255
(voice/TTY/toll-free)
www.asha.org

American Tinnitus Association (ATA)
P.O. Box 5
Portland, OR 97207-0005
800-634-8978 (toll-free)
www.ata.org

Self Help for Hard of Hearing People, Inc. (SHHH)
7910 Woodmont Avenue
Suite 1200
Bethesda, MD 20814
301-657-2248
301-657-2249 (TTY)
www.shhh.org

Laurent Clerc National Deaf Education Center
Gallaudet University
800 Florida Avenue, NE
Washington, DC 20002-3695
202-651-5000 (voice/TTY)
http://clerccenter.gallaudet.edu

For more information about health and aging, contact:
National Institute on Aging Information Center
P.O. Box 8057
Gaithersburg, MD 20898-8057
800-222-2225 (toll-free)
800-222-4225 (TTY/toll-free)

- To order publications (in English or Spanish) online, visit www.niapublications.org.
- The National Institute on Aging website is www.nia.nih.gov.
- Visit NIHSeniorHealth.gov (www.nihseniorhealth.gov), a senior-friendly website from the National Institute on Aging and the National Library of Medicine. This simple-to-use website features popular health topics for older adults. It has large type and a "talking" function that reads the text out loud.

September 2002

High Blood Pressure

You can have high blood pressure, also called *hypertension*, and still feel just fine. That's because high blood pressure does not cause symptoms that you can see or feel. But, high blood pressure, sometimes called the "silent killer," is a major health problem. If not treated, it can lead to stroke, heart disease, eye problems, or kidney failure. The good news is that there are ways you can prevent high blood pressure. And, if you already have high blood pressure, there are ways to control it and prevent its complications.

What is Blood Pressure?

When your doctor checks your blood pressure and tells you the result, she or he will say two numbers. The numbers are written one above, or before, the other. The first, or top, number is your *systolic pressure*. This tells you how much the blood flowing through your blood vessels pushes against the vessel walls as your heart beats. The second, or bottom, number measures the pressure while the heart relaxes between beats. This is the *diastolic pressure*. If your blood pressure is normal, your systolic pressure is less than 120 and your diastolic pressure is less than 80—for example, 119/79.

Do You Have High Blood Pressure?

One reason to have regular checkups by your doctor is to check your blood pressure. If you have only a slightly higher reading—such as a top number between 120 and 139 or the bottom number between 80 and 89, you have *prehypertension*. You may be at risk for developing high blood pressure. Your health care provider will probably want you to make changes in your daily habits to try and lower those numbers.

Your doctor will say your blood pressure is high when it measures 140/90 or higher at two or more checkups. He or she may also ask you to check your blood pressure at home at different times of the day. If the numbers are still high after several checks, your health care provider will probably suggest medicine, changes in your diet, and exercise.

What if Just the First Number is High?

For older people, the first number (systolic) often is high (greater than 140), but the second number (diastolic) is normal (less than 90). This problem is called *isolated systolic hypertension*. Isolated systolic hypertension is the most common form of high blood pressure in older people.

Isolated systolic hypertension can lead to serious health problems. It should be treated in the same way as regular high blood pressure. If your systolic pressure is over 140, ask your doctor how you can lower it.

Can You Prevent or Control High Blood Pressure?

More than half of Americans over age 60 have high blood pressure. But, that does not mean it is part of normal aging. Try these healthy habits to help you control or prevent high blood pressure.

Keep a healthy weight. Being overweight adds to your risk of high blood pressure. Ask your doctor if you need to lose weight.

Exercise every day. Moderate exercise can lower your risk of heart disease. Try to exercise at least 30 minutes a day, 5 days a week or more. Check with your doctor before starting a new exercise plan if you have a long-term health problem or if you are a man over 40 or a woman over 50.

Eat more fruits, vegetables, whole grains, and low-fat dairy foods. A healthy diet is important. To control high blood pressure, eat a diet rich in these foods. Make sure you are getting enough potassium. Fresh fruits and vegetables are high in potassium. If using packaged foods, read the nutrition labels to choose those that have more potassium.

Cut down on salt and sodium. Most Americans eat more salt and sodium than they need. A low-salt diet might help lower your blood pressure. Talk with your doctor about your salt intake.

Drink less alcohol. Drinking alcohol can affect your blood pressure. The effect is different depending on body size. As a general rule, men shouldn't have more than two drinks a day; women not more than one drink a day.

Follow your doctor's orders. If lifestyle changes alone do not control your high blood pressure, your doctor may tell you to take blood pressure pills. You may need to take your medicine for the rest of your life. If you have questions about it, talk to your doctor.

High Blood Pressure Facts

If you have high blood pressure, remember that:

- High blood pressure may not make you feel sick, but it is serious. See a doctor to treat it.

- You can lower your blood pressure by changing your daily habits and, if needed, by taking medicine. If you need to take high blood pressure medicine, lifestyle changes may help lower the dose you need and reduce side effects.

  - Are you already taking blood pressure medicine and your blood pressure is less than 120/80? That's good. It means the lifestyle changes and medicine are working. But if another doctor asks if you have high blood pressure, the answer is still "yes, but it is being treated."

- Tell your doctor about all the drugs you take. Don't forget to mention over-the-counter drugs, vitamins, and dietary supplements. They may affect your blood pressure. They also can change how well your blood pressure medicine works.

- Blood pressure pills should be taken at the same time each day. For example, take your medicine in the morning with breakfast or in the evening after brushing your teeth. If you miss a dose, do not double the dose the next day. Call your doctor to find out what to do.

- If you have high blood pressure, test it at home between checkups. Ask your doctor, the nurse, or your pharmacist to show you how. Make sure you are seated with your feet on the floor and your back has something to lean against. Relax quietly for five minutes before checking your blood pressure. Your arm should be resting on a support at the level of your heart. Keep a list of the results to share with the doctor, physician's assistant, or nurse.

For More Information

To learn more about high blood pressure, contact:

National Heart, Lung, and Blood Institute Health Information Center
P.O. Box 30105
Bethesda, MD 20824-0105
301-592-8573
www.nhlbi.nih.gov

National Library of Medicine MedlinePlus
www.medlineplus.gov

- In Health Topics, go to: "High Blood Pressure"

American Heart Association
7272 Greenville Avenue
Dallas, TX 75231
800-242-8721 (toll-free)
www.americanheart.org

For more information about health and aging, contact:

National Institute on Aging Information Center
P.O. Box 8057
Gaithersburg, MD 20898-8057
800-222-2225 (toll-free)
800-222-4225 (TTY/toll-free)

- To order publications (in English or Spanish) online, visit www.niapublications.org.

- The National Institute on Aging website is www.nia.nih.gov.

- Visit NIHSeniorHealth.gov (www.nihseniorhealth.gov), a senior-friendly website from the National Institute on Aging and the National Library of Medicine. This simple-to-use website features popular health topics for older adults. It has large type and a "talking" function that reads the text out loud.

July 2004

HIV, AIDS, and Older People

Grace was dating again. George, a close family friend she had known for a long time, was starting to stay overnight more and more often. Because she was past childbearing age, Grace didn't think about using condoms. And because she had known George for so long, she didn't think to ask him about his sexual history. So, Grace was shocked when she tested positive for HIV.

What is HIV? What is AIDS?

Like most people, you probably have heard a lot about HIV and AIDS. You may have thought that these diseases weren't your problem and that only younger people have to worry about them. But anyone at any age can get HIV/AIDS.

HIV (short for *human immunodeficiency virus*) is a virus that damages the immune system—the system your body uses to fight off diseases. HIV infection leads to a much more serious disease called AIDS (*acquired immunodeficiency syndrome*). When the HIV infection gets in your body, your immune system can weaken. This puts you in danger of getting other life-threatening diseases, infections, and cancers. When that happens, you have AIDS. AIDS is the last stage of HIV infection. If you think you may have HIV, it is very important to get tested. Today there are drugs that can help your body keep the HIV in check and fight against AIDS.

What Are the Symptoms of HIV/AIDS?

Many people have no symptoms when they first become infected with HIV. It can take as little as a few weeks for minor, flu-like symptoms to show up, or more than ten years for more serious symptoms to appear. Signs of HIV include headache, cough, diarrhea, swollen glands, lack of energy, loss of appetite and weight loss, fevers and sweats, repeated yeast infections, skin rashes, pelvic and abdominal cramps, sores in the mouth or on certain parts of the body, or short-term memory loss.

How Do People Get HIV and AIDS?

Anyone, at any age, can get HIV and AIDS. HIV usually comes from having unprotected sex or sharing needles with an infected person, or through contact with HIV-infected blood. No matter your age, you may be at risk if:

- *You are sexually active and do not use a latex or polyurethane condom.* You can get HIV/AIDS from having sex with someone who has HIV. The virus passes from the infected person to his or her partner in blood, semen, and vaginal fluid. During sex, HIV can get into your body through any opening, such as a

Getting Tested for HIV/AIDS

- It can take as long as 3 to 6 months after the infection for the virus to show up in your blood.

- Your health care provider can test your blood for HIV/AIDS. If you don't have a health care provider, check your local phone book for the phone number of a hospital or health center where you can get a list of test sites.

- Many health care providers who test for HIV also can provide counseling.

- In most states the tests are private, and you can choose to take the test without giving your name.

You can now also test your blood at home. The "Home Access Express HIV-1 Test System" is made by the Home Access Health Corporation. You can buy it at the drug store. It is the only HIV home test system approved by the Food and Drug Administration (FDA) and legally sold in the United States. Other HIV home test systems and kits you might see on the Internet or in magazines or newspapers have not been approved by FDA and may not always give correct results.

---

tear or cut in the lining of the vagina, vulva, penis, rectum, or mouth. Latex condoms can help prevent an infected person from transferring the HIV virus to you. (Natural condoms do not protect against HIV/AIDS as well as the latex and polyurethane types.)

- *You do not know your partner's drug and sexual history.* What you don't know can hurt you. Even though it may be hard to do, it's very important to ask your partner about his or her sexual history and drug use. Here are some questions to ask: Has your partner been tested for HIV/AIDS? Has he or she had a number of different sex partners? Has your partner ever had unprotected sex with someone who has shared needles? Has he or she injected drugs or shared needles with someone else? Drug users are not the only people who might share needles. For example, people with diabetes who inject insulin or draw blood to test glucose levels might share needles.

- *You have had a blood transfusion or operation in a developing country at any time.*

- *You had a blood transfusion in the United States between 1978 and 1985.*

Is HIV/AIDS Different in Older People?

A growing number of older people now have HIV/AIDS. About 19 percent of all people with HIV/AIDS in this country are age 50 and older. This is because doctors are finding HIV more often than ever before in older people and because improved treatments are helping people with the disease live longer.

But there may even be many more cases than we know about. Why? One reason may be that doctors do not always test older people for HIV/AIDS and so may miss some cases during routine checkups. Another may be that older people often mistake signs of HIV/AIDS for the aches and pains of normal aging, so they are less likely than younger people to get tested for the disease. Also, they may be ashamed or afraid of being tested. People age 50 and older may have the virus for years before being tested. By the time they are diagnosed with HIV/AIDS, the virus may be in the late stages.

The number of HIV/AIDS cases among older people is growing every year because:

- Older Americans know less about HIV/AIDS than younger people. They do not always know how it spreads or the importance of using condoms, not sharing needles, getting tested for HIV, and talking about it with their doctor.
- Health care workers and educators often do not talk with middle-age and older people about HIV/AIDS prevention.
- Older people are less likely than younger people to talk about their sex lives or drug use with their doctors.
- Doctors may not ask older patients about their sex lives or drug use or talk to them about risky behaviors.

Facts About HIV/AIDS

You may have read or heard things that are not true about how you get HIV/AIDS. Here are the FACTS:

- **You cannot get HIV through casual contact such as shaking hands or hugging a person with HIV/AIDS.**
- **You cannot get HIV from using a public telephone, drinking fountain, restroom, swimming pool, Jacuzzi, or hot tub.**
- **You cannot get HIV from sharing a drink.**
- **You cannot get HIV from being coughed or sneezed on by a person with HIV/AIDS.**
- **You cannot get HIV from giving blood.**
- **You cannot get HIV from a mosquito bite.**

Anyone facing a serious disease like HIV/AIDS may become very depressed. This is a special problem for older people, who may have no strong network of friends or family who can help. At the same time, they also may be coping with other diseases common to aging such as high blood pressure, diabetes, or heart problems. As the HIV/AIDS gets worse, many will need help getting around and caring for themselves. Older people with HIV/AIDS need support and understanding from their doctors, family, and friends.

HIV/AIDS can affect older people in yet another way. Many younger people who are infected turn to their parents and grandparents for financial support and nursing care. Older people who are not themselves infected by the virus may find they have to care for their own children with HIV/AIDS and then sometimes for their orphaned or HIV-infected grandchildren. Taking care of others can be mentally, physically, and financially draining. This is especially true for older caregivers. The problem becomes even worse when older caregivers have AIDS or other serious health problems. Remember, it is important to get tested for HIV/AIDS early. Early treatment increases the chances of living longer.

HIV/AIDS in People of Color and Women

The number of HIV/AIDS cases is rising in people of color across the country. About half of all people with HIV/AIDS are African American or Hispanic.

The number of cases of HIV/AIDS for women has also been growing over the past few years. The rise in the number of cases in women of color age 50 and older has been especially steep. Most got the virus from sex with infected partners. Many others got HIV through shared needles. Because women may live longer than men and because of the rising divorce rate, many widowed, divorced, and separated women are dating these days. Like older men, many older women may be at risk because they do not know how HIV/AIDS is spread. Women who no longer worry about getting pregnant may be less likely to use a condom and to practice safe sex. Also, vaginal dryness and thinning often occurs as women age; when that happens, sexual activity can lead to small cuts and tears that raise the risk for HIV/AIDS.

Treatment and Prevention

There is no cure for HIV/AIDS. But if you become infected, there are drugs that help keep the HIV virus in check and slow the spread of HIV in the body. Doctors are now using a combination of drugs called HAART (*highly active antiretroviral therapy*) to treat HIV/AIDS. Although it is not a cure, HAART is greatly reducing the number of deaths from AIDS in this country.

Prevention. Remember, there are things you can do to keep from getting HIV/AIDS. Practice the steps below to lower your risk:

- If you are having sex, make sure your partner has been tested and is free of HIV.
- Use male or female condoms (latex or polyurethane) during sexual intercourse.
- Do not share needles or any other equipment used to inject drugs.
- Get tested if you or your partner had a blood transfusion between 1978 and 1985.
- Get tested if you or your partner has had an operation or blood transfusion in a developing country at any time.

For More Information

Health agencies in most cities offer HIV testing. The following national organizations have information about HIV/AIDS:

Centers for Disease Control and Prevention (CDC)
National AIDS Hotline
800-232-4636 (toll-free)
888-232-6348 (TTY/toll-free)
www.cdc.gov

- Operated 24 hours a day, 7 days a week, in English, en Español

CDC National Prevention Information Network
P.O. Box 6003
Rockville, Maryland 20849-6003
800-458-5231 (toll-free)
800-243-7012 (TTY/toll-free)
www.cdcnpin.org

- Monday to Friday, 9 a.m. to 6 p.m. Eastern Time, in English, en Español

National Institute of Allergy and Infectious Diseases (NIAID)
Office of Communications and Public Liaison
6610 Rockledge Drive, MSC 6612
Bethesda, MD 20892-6612
301-496-5717
www.niaid.nih.gov

AIDSinfo
P.O. Box 6303
Rockville, MD 20849-6303
800-448-0440 (toll-free)
888-480-3739 (TTY/toll-free)
www.aidsinfo.nih.gov

- Monday to Friday, 12 p.m. to 5 p.m. Eastern Time, in English, en Español

National Association on HIV Over Fifty
23 Miner Street
Boston, MA 02215-3318
617-233-7107
www.hivoverfifty.org

Senior Action in a Gay Environment (SAGE)
305 7th Avenue, 16th Floor
New York, NY 10001
212-741-2247
www.sageusa.org

For more information about health and aging, contact:

National Institute on Aging Information Center
P.O. Box 8057
Gaithersburg, MD 20898-8057
800-222-2225 (toll-free)
800-222-4225 (TTY/toll-free)

- To order publications (in English or Spanish) online, visit *www.niapublications.org*.

- The National Institute on Aging website is *www.nia.nih.gov*.

- Visit NIHSeniorHealth.gov (*www.nihseniorhealth.gov*), a senior-friendly website from the National Institute on Aging and the National Library of Medicine. This simple-to-use website features popular health topics for older adults. It has large type and a "talking" function that reads the text out loud.

June 2004

Menopause

> "My mom never talked to me about menopause. She says her mother never talked about it either."
>
> "I'm not sad I'm past menopause. I'm glad those monthly periods are over."
>
> "Is it hot in here, or is it me?"

Menopause, or the "change of life," is different for each woman. For example, hot flashes and sleep problems may trouble your sister. Meanwhile, you could have a new sense of freedom and energy. Your best friend might hardly be aware of a change at all.

What is Menopause?

Menopause is a normal part of life, just like puberty. It is the time of your last period, but symptoms can begin several years before that. And these symptoms can last for months or years after. Some time around 40, you might notice that your period is different—how long it lasts, how much you bleed, or how often it happens may not be the same. Or, without warning, you might find yourself feeling very warm during the day or in the middle of the night. Changing levels of estrogen and progesterone, which are two female hormones made in your ovaries, might lead to these symptoms.

This time of change, called *perimenopause* by many women and their doctors, often begins several years before your last menstrual period. It lasts for 1 year after your last period, the point in time known as *menopause*. A full year without a period is needed before you can say you have been "through menopause." *Postmenopause* follows menopause and lasts the rest of your life.

Menopause doesn't usually happen before you are 40, but it can happen any time from your 30s to your mid 50s or later. The average age is 51. Smoking can lead to early menopause. Some types of surgery can bring on menopause. For example, removing your uterus (hysterectomy) before menopause will make your periods stop, but your ovaries will still make hormones. That means you could still have symptoms of menopause like hot flashes when your ovaries start to make less estrogen. But, when both ovaries are also removed (oophorectomy), menopause symptoms can start right away, no matter what your age is, because your body has lost its main supply of estrogen.

What Are the Signs of Menopause?

Women may have different signs or symptoms at menopause. That's because estrogen is used by many parts of your body. So, changes in how much estrogen you have can cause assorted symptoms. But, that doesn't mean you will have all, or even most, of them. In fact, some of the signs that happen around the time of menopause may really be a result of growing older, not changes in estrogen.

Changes in your period. This might be what you notice first. Your period may no longer be regular. How much you bleed could change. It could be lighter than normal. Or, you could have a heavier flow. Periods may be shorter or last longer. These are all normal results of changes in your reproductive system as you grow older. But, just to make sure there isn't a problem, see your doctor if:

- Your periods are coming very close together,
- You have heavy bleeding,
- You have spotting, or
- Your periods are lasting more than a week.

Hot flashes. These are very common around the time of menopause because they are related to changing estrogen levels. These may last a few years after menopause. A *hot flash* is a sudden feeling of heat in the upper part or all of your body. Your face and neck become flushed. Red blotches may appear on your chest, back, and arms. Heavy sweating and cold shivering can follow. Flashes can be as mild as a light blush or severe enough to wake you from a sound sleep (called *night sweats*). Most hot flashes last between 30 seconds and 10 minutes.

Problems with the vagina and bladder. Changing estrogen levels can cause your genital area to get drier and thinner. This could make sexual intercourse uncomfortable. You could have more vaginal or urinary infections. You might find it hard to hold urine long enough to get to the bathroom. Sometimes your urine might leak during exercise, sneezing, coughing, laughing, or running.

Sex. Around the time of menopause you may find that your feelings about sex have changed. You could be less interested. Or, you could feel freer and sexier after menopause. You can stop worrying about becoming pregnant after one full year without a period. But, remember you can't ever stop worrying about sexually-transmitted diseases (STDs), such as HIV/AIDS or gonorrhea. If you think you might be at risk for an STD, make sure your partner uses a condom each time you have sex.

Sleep problems. You might start having trouble getting a good night's sleep. Maybe

MENOPAUSE 39

you can't fall asleep easily, or you wake too early. Night sweats might wake you up. You might have trouble falling back to sleep if you wake during the night.

Mood changes. You might find yourself more moody, irritable, or depressed around the time of menopause. It's not clear why this happens—is there is a connection between changes in estrogen levels and emotions or not? It's possible that stress, family changes such as growing children or aging parents, or always feeling tired could be causing these mood changes.

Changes in your body. You might think your body is changing. Your waist could get larger. You could lose muscle and gain fat. Your skin could get thinner. You might have memory problems, and your joints and muscles could feel stiff and achy. Are these a result of having less estrogen or just related to growing older? We don't know.

What About My Heart and Bones?

Two common health problems can start to happen at menopause, and you might not even notice.

Osteoporosis. Day in and day out your body is busy breaking down old bone and replacing it with new healthy bone. Estrogen helps control bone loss. So losing estrogen around the time of menopause causes women to begin to lose more bone than is replaced. In time, bones can become weak and break easily. This condition is called osteoporosis. Talk to your doctor to see if you should have a bone density test to find out if you are at risk for this problem. Your doctor can also suggest ways to prevent or treat osteoporosis.

Heart disease. After menopause, women are more likely to have heart disease. Changes in estrogen levels may be part of the cause. But, so is getting older. As you age, you may develop other problems, like high blood pressure or weight gain, that put you at greater risk for heart disease. Be sure to have your blood pressure and levels of triglycerides, fasting blood glucose, and LDL, HDL, and total cholesterol checked regularly. Talk to your health care provider to find out what you should do to protect your heart.

How Can I Stay Healthy After Menopause?

Staying healthy after menopause may mean making some changes in the way you live.

- Don't smoke. If you do use any type of tobacco, stop—it's never too late to benefit from quitting smoking.

- Eat a healthy diet—one low in fat, high in fiber, with plenty of fruits, vegetables, and whole-grain foods, as well as all the important vitamins and minerals.

- Make sure you get enough calcium and vitamin D—in your diet or in vitamin and mineral supplements.
- Learn what your healthy weight is, and try to stay there.
- Do weight-bearing exercise, such as walking, jogging, or dancing at least 3 days each week for healthy bones. But try to be physically active in other ways for your general health.

Other things to remember:

- Take medicine to lower your blood pressure if your doctor prescribes it for you.
- Use a water-based vaginal lubricant (*not* petroleum jelly) or a vaginal estrogen cream or tablet to help with vaginal discomfort.
- Get regular pelvic and breast exams, Pap tests, and mammograms. You should also be checked for colon and rectal cancer and for skin cancer. Contact your doctor right away if you notice a lump in your breast or a mole that has changed.

Are you bothered by hot flashes? Menopause is not a disease that has to be treated. But you might need help with symptoms like hot flashes. Here are some ideas that have helped some women:

- Try to keep track of when hot flashes happen—a diary can help. You might be able to use this information to find out what triggers your flashes and then avoid it.
- When a hot flash starts, go somewhere cool.
- If night sweats wake you, try sleeping in a cool room or with a fan on.
- Dress in layers that you can take off if you get too warm.
- Use sheets and clothing that let your skin "breathe."
- Have a cold drink (water or juice) when a flash is starting.

You could also talk to your doctor about whether there are any medicines to manage hot flashes. Gabapentin, megestrol acetate, and certain antidepressants seem to be helpful to some women.

What About Those Lost Hormones?

These days you hear a lot about whether you should use hormones to help relieve some menopause symptoms. It's hard to know what to do.

During perimenopause, some doctors suggest birth control pills to help with very heavy, frequent, or unpredictable menstrual periods. These pills might also help with symptoms like hot flashes, as well as prevent pregnancy.

As you get closer to menopause, you might be bothered more by symptoms like hot flashes, night sweats, or vaginal dryness. Your doctor might then suggest

MENOPAUSE 41

taking estrogen (as well as progesterone, if you still have a uterus). This is known as *menopausal hormone therapy (MHT)*. Some people still call it hormone replacement therapy or HRT. Taking these hormones will probably help with menopause symptoms and prevent the bone loss that can happen at menopause. However, there is a chance your symptoms will come back when you stop MHT.

Also, menopausal hormone therapy has risks. That is why the U.S. Food and Drug Administration suggests that women who want to try MHT to manage their hot flashes or vaginal dryness use the lowest dose that works for the shortest time it's needed.

Right now, there is a lot that is unknown about taking hormones around menopause. Use the resource listing at the end of this *Age Page* if you would like to learn more about menopause or if you want the latest information on menopausal hormone therapy.

Do Phytoestrogens Help?

Phytoestrogens are estrogen-like substances found in some cereals, vegetables, legumes (beans), and herbs. They might work in the body like a weak form of estrogen. They might relieve some symptoms of menopause, but they could also carry risks like estrogen. We don't know. Be sure to tell your doctor if you decide to try eating a lot more foods that contain phytoestrogens or to try using an herbal supplement. Any food or over-the-counter product that you use for its drug-like effects could change how other prescribed drugs work or cause an overdose.

How Do I Decide What to Do?

Talk to your health care provider for help deciding how to best manage menopause. You can see a gynecologist, geriatrician, general practitioner, or internist. Talk about your symptoms and whether they bother you. Make sure the doctor knows your medical history and your family medical history. This includes whether you are at risk for heart disease, osteoporosis, and breast cancer. Remember that your decision is never final. You can—and should—review it with your doctor during a checkup. Your needs may change, and so might what we know about menopause.

A hundred years ago life expectancy was a lot shorter. Reaching menopause then often meant that a woman's life was nearing its end. Not so now. Women are living much longer. Today, a woman turning 50 can expect to live, on average, almost 32 more years. You have the time and freedom to make them active, busy years. Follow a healthy lifestyle and plan to make the most of those years ahead of you!

For More Information

For more detailed answers to your questions about menopause, contact:

National Institutes of Health Menopausal Hormone Therapy Information
www.nih.gov/PHTindex.htm

National Library of Medicine MedlinePlus
www.medlineplus.gov

- In Health Topics, go to: "Menopause"

American College of Obstetricians and Gynecologists
409 12th Street, SW
P.O. Box 96920
Washington, DC 20090
202-638-5577
www.acog.org

North American Menopause Society
P.O. Box 94527
Cleveland, OH 44101
440-442-7550
www.menopause.org

For more information on health and aging, including menopausal hormone therapy and osteoporosis, contact:

National Institute on Aging Information Center
P.O. Box 8057
Gaithersburg, MD 20898-8057
800-222-2225 (toll-free)
800-222-4225 (TTY/toll-free)

- To order publications (in English or Spanish) online, visit *www.niapublications.org*.
- The National Institute on Aging website is *www.nia.nih.gov*.
- Visit NIHSeniorHealth.gov (*www.nihseniorhealth.gov*), a senior-friendly website from the National Institute on Aging and the National Library of Medicine. This simple-to-use website features popular health topics for older adults. It has large type and a "talking" function that reads the text out loud.

June 2005

Osteoporosis: The Bone Thief

> Helen grew up on a farm in the Midwest. She drank lots of milk as a child. She also walked a lot. After graduating from high school, she got married and found a job. Family and work kept her too busy to exercise. Helen went through menopause at age 47. At age 76, she was enjoying retirement—traveling and working in her garden. But then she slipped on a small rug in her kitchen and broke her hip. After Helen recovered, she needed a cane to walk, and gardening was a lot harder to enjoy.

Helen had *osteoporosis*, but she didn't know it before she fell. Osteoporosis is a disease that weakens bones to the point where they break easily—most often bones in the hip, backbone (spine), and wrist. Osteoporosis is called the "silent disease"—you may not notice any changes until a bone breaks. But your bones have been losing strength for many years.

Bone is living tissue. To keep bones strong, your body is always breaking down old bone and replacing it with new bone tissue. As people enter their forties and fifties, more bone is broken down than is replaced. A close look at the inside of bone shows something like a honeycomb. When you have osteoporosis, the spaces in this honeycomb grow larger. And the bone that forms the honeycomb gets smaller. The outer shell of your bones also gets thinner. All this loss makes your bones weaker.

Who Has Osteoporosis?

Millions of Americans have osteoporosis. They are mostly women, but more than two million men also have this disease. White and Asian women are most likely to have osteoporosis. Other women at great risk include those who:

- Have a family history of the disease,
- Have broken a bone while an adult,
- Had surgery to remove their ovaries before their periods stopped,
- Had early menopause,
- Have not gotten enough calcium throughout their lives,
- Had extended bed rest,
- Used certain medicines for a long time, or
- Have a small body frame.

The risk of osteoporosis grows as you get older. At the time of menopause women may lose bone quickly for several years. After that, the loss slows down, but continues. In men the loss of bone mass is slower. But, by age 65 or 70 men and women are losing bone at the same rate.

What is Osteopenia?

Millions more Americans have *osteopenia*. Whether your doctor calls it osteopenia or just says you have low bone mass, consider it a warning. Bone loss has started, but you can still take action to keep your bones strong and maybe prevent osteoporosis later in life. That way you will be less likely to break a wrist, hip, or vertebrae (bone in your spine) when you are older.

Can My Bones be Tested?

For some people the first sign of osteoporosis is to realize they are getting shorter or to break a bone easily, like Helen. Don't wait until that happens to see if you have osteoporosis. You can have a *bone density* test to find out how solid your bones are. Your doctor may suggest a type of bone density test called a DEXA-scan (dual-energy x-ray absorptiometry) if you are age 65 or older or if he or she thinks you are at risk for osteoporosis.

The DEXA-scan tells what your risk for a fracture or broken bone is. It could show that you have normal bone density. Or, it could show that you have low bone mass or even osteoporosis.

How Can I Keep My Bones Strong?

There are things you should do at any age to prevent weakened bones. Eating foods that are rich in calcium and vitamin D is important. So is including regular weight-bearing exercise in your lifestyle. These are the best ways to keep your bones strong and healthy.

Calcium. Getting enough calcium all through your life helps to build and keep strong bones. People over age 50 need 1,200 mg of calcium every day. Foods that are high in calcium are the best source. For example, eat low-fat dairy foods, canned fish with soft bones such as salmon, dark green leafy vegetables, and calcium-fortified foods like orange juice, breads, and cereals.

If you think you aren't getting enough calcium in your diet, check with your doctor first. He or she may tell you to try a calcium supplement. Calcium carbonate and calcium citrate are two common forms. You have to be careful though. Too much calcium can cause problems for some people. On most days you should not get more than 2,500 mg of total calcium. That includes calcium from all sources—foods, drinks, and supplements.

Vitamin D. Your body uses vitamin D to absorb calcium. Most people's bodies are able to make enough vitamin D if they are out in the sun for a total of 20 minutes every day. You can also get vitamin D from eggs, fatty fish, and cereal and milk fortified with vitamin D. If you think you are not getting enough vitamin D, check with your doctor. Each day you should have:

- 400 IU (international unit) if you are age 51–70, or
- 600 IU if you are over age 70.

As with calcium, be careful. More than 2,000 IU of vitamin D each day may cause side effects.

Exercise. Your bones and muscles will be stronger if you are physically active. Weight-bearing exercises, done three to four times a week, are best for preventing osteoporosis. Walking, jogging, playing tennis, and dancing are examples of weight-bearing exercises. Try some strengthening and balance exercises, too. They may help you avoid falls which could cause a broken bone.

Medicines. Some common medicines can make bones weaker. These include a type of steroid drug called glucocorticoids used for arthritis and asthma, some antiseizure drugs, certain sleeping pills, treatments for endometriosis, and some cancer drugs. An overactive thyroid gland or using too much thyroid hormone for an underactive thyroid can also be a problem. If you are taking these medicines, talk to your doctor about what you can do to help protect your bones.

Lifestyle. Smoking increases loss of bone mass. For this and many other health reasons, stop smoking. Limit how much alcohol you drink. Too much alcohol can put you at risk for falling and breaking a bone.

What Can I Do for My Osteoporosis?

Treating osteoporosis means stopping the bone loss and rebuilding bone to prevent breaks. Diet and exercise can help make your bones stronger. But they may not be enough if you have lost a lot of bone density. There are also several medicines to think about. Some will slow your bone loss, and others can help rebuild bone. Talk with your doctor to see if one of these might work for you:

- *Alendronate or risedronate.* These medicines are bisphosphonates, drugs that slow the breakdown of bone and increase bone density. They can make it less likely that you will break a bone, most of all in your spine, hip, or wrist. Side effects may include nausea, heartburn, and stomach pain. A few people have muscle, bone, or joint pain while using these medicines. These drugs must be taken in a certain way— when you first get up, before you have eaten, **and** with a full glass of water. You **should not** lie down, eat, or drink for at least one-half hour after taking the drug. Even if you follow the directions closely, these drugs can cause serious digestive problems so be aware of any side effects. These pills are available in both once-daily and once-a-week versions.

- *Raloxifene.* This drug is used to prevent and treat osteoporosis. It is a SERM (selective estrogen receptor modulator). It prevents bone loss and spine fractures, but may cause hot flashes or increase the risk of blood clots in some women.

- *Estrogen.* Doctors sometimes prescribe this female hormone around the time of menopause to treat symptoms like hot flashes or vaginal dryness. Estrogen also slows bone loss and increases bone mass in your spine and hip, so women can use it to prevent or treat osteoporosis. But, estrogen use is thought to be risky for some women. Talk to your doctor. Ask about the benefits, risks, and side effects, as well as other possible treatments for you.

- *Calcitonin.* This hormone increases bone mass in your spine and can lessen the pain of fractures already there. It comes in two forms—a shot or nasal spray. The shot may cause an allergic reaction and has some side effects like nausea, diarrhea, or redness in your face, ears, hands, or feet. The only side effect of the nasal spray is a runny nose in some people. Calcitonin is most useful for women who are five years past menopause.

- *Parathyroid hormone (PTH).* Also called teriparatide, this shot is given daily for up to two years to postmenopausal women and men who are at high risk for broken bones. It improves bone density in the spine and hip. Common side effects include nausea, dizziness, and leg cramps.

Can I Avoid Falling?

When your bones are weak, a simple fall can cause a broken bone. This can mean a trip to the hospital and maybe surgery. It might also mean being laid up for a long time, especially in the case of a hip fracture. So, it is important to prevent falls. Some things you can do are:

- Make sure you can see and hear well. Use your glasses or a hearing aid if needed.
- Ask your doctor if any of the drugs you are taking can make you dizzy or unsteady on your feet.
- Use a cane or walker if your walking is unsteady.
- Wear rubber-soled and low-heeled shoes.
- Make sure all the rugs and carpeting in your house are firmly attached to the floor, or don't use them.
- Keep your rooms well lit and the floor free of clutter.
- Use nightlights.

You can find more suggestions in the National Institute on Aging's *Preventing Falls and Fractures Age Page*, available from the National Institute on Aging Information Center.

Do Men Have Osteoporosis?

Osteoporosis is not just a woman's disease. Not as many men have it as women do, but men need to worry about it as well. This may be because most men start with more bone density than women and lose it more slowly as they grow older.

Experts don't know as much about this disease in men as they do in women. However, many of the things that put men at risk are the same as those for women:

- Family history,
- Not enough calcium or vitamin D,

- Too little exercise,
- Low levels of testosterone,
- Too much alcohol,
- Taking certain drugs, or
- Smoking.

Older men who break a bone easily or are at risk for osteoporosis should talk with their doctors about testing and treatment. Men can use alendronate, risedronate, or parathyroid hormone to increase bone density. Testosterone supplements may help some men with low levels of testosterone.

For More Information

The organizations listed below offer more information about some of the topics mentioned in this fact sheet:

National Osteoporosis Foundation
1232 22nd Street, NW
Washington, DC 20037-1292
202-223-2226
www.nof.org

National Institutes of Health Osteoporosis and Related Bone Diseases~National Resource Center
2 AMS Circle
Bethesda, MD 20892-3676
800-624-2663 (toll-free)
202-466-4315 (TTY)
www.osteo.org

National Library of Medicine MedlinePlus
www.medlineplus.gov
- In Health Topics, go to:
  "Osteoporosis"
  "Falls"

The National Institute on Aging has information on health and aging, including a booklet and video about exercise for older people and several helpful *Age Pages*. Contact:

National Institute on Aging Information Center
P.O. Box 8057
Gaithersburg, MD 20898-8057
800-222-2225 (toll-free)
800-222-4225 (TTY/toll-free)

- To order publications (in English or Spanish) online, visit www.niapublications.org.

- The National Institute on Aging website is www.nia.nih.gov.
- Visit NIHSeniorHealth.gov (www.nihseniorhealth.gov), a senior-friendly website from the National Institute on Aging and the National Library of Medicine. This simple-to-use website features popular health topics for older adults. It has large type and a "talking" function that reads the text out loud.

December 2004

Prostate Problems

The prostate is a small organ about the size of a walnut. It is found below the bladder (where urine is stored) and surrounds the tube that carries urine away from the bladder (urethra). The prostate makes a fluid that becomes part of semen. Semen is the white fluid that contains sperm.

Prostate problems are common in men age 50 and older. Sometimes men feel symptoms themselves, or sometimes their doctors find prostate problems during routine exams. Doctors who are experts in diseases of the urinary tract (urologists) diagnose and treat prostate problems.

There are many different kinds of prostate problems. Many don't involve cancer, but some do. Treatments vary, but prostate problems can often be treated without affecting sexual function.

Common Problems

There are several common prostate problems including:

Acute prostatitis is an infection of the prostate caused by bacteria. It usually starts fast and can cause fever, chills, or pain in the lower back and between the legs. It also can cause pain when you urinate. If you have these symptoms, see your doctor right away. Antibiotic drugs usually help heal the infection and relieve the symptoms. Your doctor also may suggest that you drink more liquids.

Chronic prostatitis is a prostate infection that keeps coming back time after time. Symptoms may be milder than in acute prostatitis, but they can last longer. Chronic prostatitis can be hard to treat. Antibiotics may work if bacteria are causing the infection. But if bacteria are not the cause, antibiotics won't work. Massaging the prostate sometimes helps to release fluids. Warm baths also may bring relief. Often chronic prostatitis clears up by itself.

Benign prostatic hyperplasia (BPH) is the term used to describe an enlarged prostate. BPH is common in older men. Over time, an enlarged prostate may block the urethra, making it hard to urinate. It may cause dribbling after you urinate or a frequent urge to urinate, especially at night. Your doctor will conduct a rectal exam to diagnose BPH. The doctor also may look at your urethra, prostate, and bladder.

Treatment choices for BPH include:

- *Watchful waiting.* If your symptoms are not troubling, your doctor may suggest that you wait before starting any treatment. In that case, you will need regular checkups to make sure the condition does not get worse.
- *Alpha-blockers* (some generic names are doxasozin, terazosin) are medicines that can relax muscles near the prostate and ease symptoms. Side effects may include headaches, dizziness, or feeling lightheaded or tired.

- *Finasteride* (Proscar) acts on the male hormone (testosterone) to shrink the prostate. Side effects of this medication can include less interest in sex and problems with erection or ejaculation.
- *Surgery* also can relieve symptoms. But surgery can cause complications. Also, it does not protect against prostate cancer. Talk with your doctor about this treatment choice. Regular checkups are important even for men who have had BPH surgery.

There are three kinds of surgery:

- *Transurethral resection* of the prostate (TURP) is the most common type of surgery. While the patient is under anesthesia, the doctor uses a special device to take out part of the prostate and remove the blockage.
- *Transurethral incision* of the prostate (TUIP) may be used when the prostate is not too enlarged. The doctor makes a few small cuts in the prostate near the opening of the bladder. This relaxes the bladder muscles and improves the flow of urine.
- *Open surgery* is used when the prostate is very enlarged. In this process, prostate tissue is removed directly rather than through the urethra.

Prostate Cancer

Prostate cancer is one of the most common types of cancer among American men. It is more common among African American men than white men. Treatment for prostate cancer works best when the disease is found early.

Diagnosing Prostate Cancer

Doctors will ask questions about your medical history and perform a physical exam to find the cause of prostate problems. In the exam, the doctor feels the prostate through the rectal wall. Hard or lumpy areas may mean that cancer is present.

Your doctor also may suggest a blood test to check your prostate specific antigen (PSA) level. PSA levels may be high in men who have an enlarged prostate gland or prostate cancer. PSA tests are very useful for early cancer diagnosis. But PSA test results alone do not always tell whether or not cancer is present.

When doctors suspect cancer, they also may perform a biopsy. Using this simple method, doctors can take out a small piece of the prostate and look at it under a microscope.

Prostate Cancer Treatment

There are many options for treating prostate cancer. Each treatment plan is based on details, such as whether or not the cancer has spread beyond the prostate (stage of cancer), your age and general health, and how you feel about the treatment options and side effects. Some of the treatment choices include:

Watchful waiting. As with BPH, if the cancer is slow growing and not causing problems, you may decide not to have treatment right away. Instead, your doctor will watch closely for changes in your condition. Men who are older or have another serious illness often choose this option.

Surgery is used to take out the cancer. Among the different types of surgery for prostate cancer are:

- *Radical prostatectomy.* This surgery takes out the entire prostate and nearby tissues. Side effects may include lack of sexual function (impotence) or problems holding urine (incontinence). Improvements in surgery now make it possible for some men to keep their sexual function. Some men with trouble holding urine may regain control within several weeks of surgery. Others continue to have problems that require them to wear a pad.
- *Cryosurgery* kills the cancer by freezing it.

Radiation therapy uses high-energy X-rays to kill cancer cells and shrink tumors. Radiation therapy sometimes is beamed into the prostate from outside the body. It can cause problems with impotence and bowel function.

- *Brachytherapy* is a type of radiation therapy often used when the cancer is found only in the prostate gland. It also is sometimes called internal radiation, implant radiation, or interstitial radiation therapy. In this treatment, the doctor places radioactive "seeds" directly into the prostate. This focuses the radiation directly on the cancer and lowers the chance of affecting other, healthy areas around the prostate.

Hormone therapy stops cancer cells from growing. The growth of prostate cancer often depends on testosterone. Drug treatment is one effective way to block testosterone. This treatment is often used for prostate cancer that has spread to other parts of the body.

You can get more detailed information on the pros and cons of these treatment choices by calling the National Cancer Institute's Cancer Information Service at 800-422-6237. Ask for prostate cancer information in "PDQ for Patients."

Protecting Yourself

These are the signs of prostate problems:

- Frequent urge to urinate,
- Blood in urine or semen,
- Painful or burning urination,
- Difficulty in urinating,
- Difficulty in having an erection,
- Painful ejaculation,
- Frequent pain or stiffness in lower back, hips, or upper thighs,
- Inability to urinate, or
- Dribbling of urine.

If you have any of these symptoms, see your doctor right away to find out if you need treatment.

For More Information

More information on prostate problems is available from:

National Cancer Institute
Cancer Information Service
800-422-6237 (toll-free)
800-332-8615 (TTY/toll-free)
www.cancer.gov

National Institute of Diabetes and Digestive and Kidney Diseases
National Kidney and Urological Diseases Information Clearinghouse
3 Information Way
Bethesda, MD 20892-3580
800-891-5390 (toll-free)
301-654-4415
www.niddk.nih.gov

Agency for Healthcare Research & Quality
Publications Clearinghouse
P.O. Box 8547
Silver Spring, MD 20907-8547
800-358-9295 (toll-free)
www.ahrq.gov

American Cancer Society
1599 Clifton Road, NE
Atlanta, GA 30329
800-227-2345 (toll-free)
404-320-3333
www.cancer.org

American Urological Association Foundation, Inc.
1000 Corporate Boulevard
Linthicum, MD 21090
866-746-4282 (toll-free)
410-689-3700
www.urologyhealth.org

For more information about health and aging, contact:
National Institute on Aging Information Center
P.O. Box 8057
Gaithersburg, MD 20898-8057
800-222-2225 (toll-free)
800-222-4225 (TTY/toll-free)

- To order publications (in English or Spanish) online, visit www.niapublications.org.
- The National Institute on Aging website is www.nia.nih.gov.
- Visit NIHSeniorHealth.gov (www.nihseniorhealth.gov), a senior-friendly website from the National Institute on Aging and the National Library of Medicine. This simple-to-use website features popular health topics for older adults. It has large type and a "talking" function that reads the text out loud.

January 2002

Shingles

> Ruth, a 79-year-old woman, said her case of shingles was causing her so much pain she couldn't bear to put on her clothes or have sheets touch her skin. Ruth was sick for several months. Her friend, Sarah, had it easier. Shingles made Sarah feel sick for a few days, and she had some discomfort. But she was back to her old self in a few weeks. Sarah noted, "Having shingles wasn't so bad."

What is Shingles?

Shingles is a disease that affects nerves and causes pain and blisters in adults. It is caused by the same varicella-zoster virus that causes chickenpox. After you recover from chickenpox, the virus does not leave your body, but continues to live in some nerve cells. For reasons that aren't totally understood, the virus can become active instead of remaining inactive. When it's activated, it produces shingles.

Just like chickenpox, people with shingles will feel sick and have a rash on their body or face. The major difference is that chickenpox is a childhood illness, while shingles targets older people. Most adults live with the virus in their body and never get shingles. But about one in five people who have had chickenpox will get shingles later in life—usually after the age of 50.

When the activated virus travels along the path of a nerve to the surface of the skin, a rash will appear. It usually shows up as a band on one side of the face or body. The word "shingles" comes from the Latin word for belt or girdle because often the rash is shaped like a belt.

Who is at Risk?

People with the varicella-zoster virus in their body can be at risk for getting shingles.

Right now there is no way of knowing who will get the disease. But, there are things that make you more likely to get shingles.

- *Advanced age.* The risk of getting shingles increases as you age. People have a hard time fighting off infections as they get older. The chance of getting shingles becomes much higher by age 70.
- *Trouble fighting infections.* Your immune system is the part of your body that fights off infections. Age can affect your immune system. So can an HIV infection, cancer, cancer drugs, radiation treatments, or organ transplant. Even stress or a cold can weaken your immune system for a short time and put you at risk for shingles.

What Are the Symptoms of Shingles?

Most people have some of the following symptoms.

- Burning, tingling, or numbness of the skin,
- Feeling sick—chills, fever, upset stomach, or headache,
- Fluid-filled blisters,
- Skin that is sensitive to touch, or
- Mild itching to strong pain.

Shingles follows a pattern. A few days after the tingling or burning feeling on the skin, a red rash will come out on your body, face, or neck. In a few days, the rash will turn into fluid-filled blisters. The blisters dry up and crust over within several days. The rash usually happens on one side of the body. Most cases of shingles last from 3–5 weeks.

Do You Need a Doctor?

George, age 67, had a red rash on his face and felt sick. His wife urged him to see a doctor, but he told her, "It's just a rash. I'll be all right in a few days." His wife insisted that he go to the doctor. The doctor told George that he had shingles and ordered some medicine for him.

It's important to go to your doctor no later than three days after the rash starts. The doctor needs to see the rash to confirm what you have and make a treatment plan. Although there is no cure for shingles, early treatment with drugs that fight the virus can help. Shingles can often be treated at home. Patients with shingles rarely need to stay in a hospital.

How is Shingles Treated?

For people with severe symptoms, there are many medications your doctor can prescribe to treat shingles. These include medicines that:

- Fight the virus—antiviral drugs,
- Lessen pain and shorten the time you're sick—steroids,
- Help with pain relief antidepressants and anticonvulsants, or
- Reduce pain—analgesics.

When started within 72 hours of getting the rash, these medicines help shorten the length of the infection and lower the risk of other problems.

Why Does the Pain Go On and On?

After the rash goes away, some people may be left with long lasting pain called post-herpetic neuralgia or PHN. The pain is felt in the same area where the rash had been. For some people, PHN is the longest lasting and worst part of shingles. The pain can make some people feel weak and unable to do things they usually enjoy. Those who have had PHN say the pain is sharp, throbbing, or stabbing. Their skin is so sensitive they can't bear to wear even soft, light clothing. People who have PHN call it a pain that won't go away.

The older you are when you get shingles, the greater your chance of developing PHN. This pain can last for weeks, months, or even years.

"I've had post-herpetic neuralgia for nine months," said Pete, an 80-year-old man. "I've lost 20 pounds. I can't find anything that helps with the pain."

The PHN pain can cause depression, anxiety, sleeplessness, and weight loss. Some people with PHN find it hard to go about their daily activities like dressing, cooking, and eating. Talk to your doctor if you have any of these problems. There are medicines that may help. Usually PHN will get better over time.

What Are Other Complications?

In some cases, blisters can become infected. Scarring of the skin may result. Your doctor can prescribe an antibiotic treatment. Keep the area clean, and try not to scratch!

There are other problems to watch for. If blisters occur near or in the eye, lasting eye damage or blindness may result. This can be very serious. See an eye doctor right away.

Other problems may include hearing loss or a brief paralysis of the face. In a small number of cases, swelling of the brain (encephalitis) can occur. It's very important to go to the doctor as soon as possible—especially if you have blisters on your face.

Can You Catch Shingles?

No, shingles is not contagious. You can't catch shingles from someone who has it. But you can catch chickenpox from someone with shingles. So, if you've never had chickenpox, try to stay away from anyone who has shingles.

Flo, a 77-year-old woman notes, "My daughter stayed away when I had shingles. She'd never had chickenpox and didn't want to risk catching it. Good thing my sister lived nearby and could help me during those first few weeks."

Will Shingles Return?

Most people get shingles only once. But it is possible to have it more than once.

What Can You Do?

If you have shingles, here are some things that may make you feel better:

- Make sure you get enough rest, avoid stress as much as you can, and eat well-balanced meals.
- Simple exercises like stretching or walking can help. Check with your doctor first.
- Dip a washcloth in cool water and apply it to your blisters to ease the pain and help dry the blisters.

SHINGLES 55

- Do things that take your mind off your pain. Watch TV, read interesting books, talk with friends, or work on a hobby you like.
- Try to relax. Stress can make the pain worse. Listen to music that helps you relax.
- Share your feelings about your pain with family and friends. Ask for their help.

What's in the Future?

The Shingles Prevention Study (SPS) is a five-year nationwide study of an experimental vaccine to prevent shingles. This vaccine is similar to the vaccine that children have been receiving since 1995 to prevent chickenpox. Scientists hope that the adult vaccine to prevent shingles will be offered in the future.

For More Information

For more information about shingles and pain management, you can call or write:

National Institute of Allergy and Infectious Diseases
6610 Rockledge Drive MSC 6612
Bethesda, MD 20892
301-496-5717
www.niaid.nih.gov

National Institute of Neurological Disorders and Stroke
P.O. Box 5801
Bethesda, MD 20824
800-352-9424 (toll-free)
301-468-5981 (TTY)
www.ninds.nih.gov

American Chronic Pain Association
P.O. Box 850
Rocklin, CA 95677-0850
800-533-3231 (toll-free)
www.theacpa.org

National Chronic Pain Outreach Association
P.O. Box 274
Millboro, VA 24460
540-862-9437
www.chronicpain.org

National Foundation for the Treatment of Pain
P.O. Box 70045
Houston, TX 77270-0045
713-862-9332
www.paincare.org

VZV Research Foundation
40 East 72nd Street
New York, NY 10021
800-472-8478 (toll-free)
www.vzvfoundation.org

For more information about health and aging, contact:

National Institute on Aging Information Center
P.O. Box 8057
Gaithersburg, MD 20898-8057
800-222-2225 (toll-free)
800-222-4225 (TTY/toll-free)

- To order publications (in English or Spanish) online, visit www.niapublications.org.
- The National Institute on Aging website is www.nia.nih.gov.
- Visit NIHSeniorHealth.gov (www.nihseniorhealth.gov), a senior-friendly website from the National Institute on Aging and the National Library of Medicine. This simple-to-use website features popular health topics for older adults. It has large type and a "talking" function that reads the text out loud.

June 2004

Stroke

> John and Edith were eating dinner one night when John asked Edith a question. She began to answer, but couldn't speak. John knew something was very wrong. Could Edith have had a stroke? Without waiting, he called 911. The ambulance took Edith to the hospital right away. Emergency room doctors confirmed John's fear…it was a stroke. But because of John's quick action in calling for help, Edith got the medical care she needed without delay. She got well quickly, her speech came back, and she's once again having long talks with John at dinner.

Edith was lucky. Stroke is the third leading cause of death in the United States after heart disease and cancer. It is a major cause of physical and mental disabilities in older adults. And every year, more and more people are affected when they or someone they know has a stroke.

What is a Stroke?

A stroke happens when blood can't flow to a part of the brain. When the brain doesn't get the oxygen and nutrients it needs from the blood, its cells are damaged or begin to die. If brain cells are only hurt, they sometimes can be repaired. But brain cells that have died can't be brought back to life. This means that the brain may stop sending signals to other parts of the body that control things like speaking, thinking, and walking.

There are two major types of strokes. The most common kind (*ischemic*) is caused by blood clots or the narrowing of a blood vessel (artery) leading to the brain. The clot keeps blood from flowing into other regions of the brain and prevents needed oxygen and nutrients from reaching brain cells in these regions. The second major kind of stroke (*hemorrhagic*) happens when a broken blood vessel (artery) causes bleeding in the brain. This break also stops oxygen and nutrients from reaching brain cells.

Stroke is an Emergency. Call 911.

Never ignore the warning signs of stroke. The warning signs of a stroke may last only a few minutes and then go away. When this happens, it could be a *mini-stroke,* which is called a TIA (*transient ischemic attack*).

This is also a medical emergency that requires attention right away. An unrecognized and untreated TIA can be followed within hours by a major disabling stroke. Always pay attention to **any** stroke symptoms, even if they are fleeting.

Call 911 RIGHT AWAY if you see or have any of these warning signs:

- Sudden *numbness or weakness* in the face, arm, or leg—especially on one side of the body,

- Sudden *confusion, trouble speaking or understanding,*

- Sudden *problems seeing* in one eye or both eyes,

- Sudden *dizziness, loss of balance or coordination,* or *trouble walking,*

- Sudden *severe headache* with no known cause.

DON'T IGNORE THE SIGNS!

What If *Is* a Stroke?

Recovery from a stroke is most successful if treatment begins within the first three hours after symptoms appear. The clot-busting drug t-PA can greatly lower the damage caused by a stroke, but it must be given within the three hour time frame. Getting to the hospital as soon as possible allows time for a CT scan of the brain. This scan will show whether t-PA is the right treatment. Only patients with ischemic stroke, caused by a clot, are candidates for this treatment. The doctor will diagnose stroke based on the patient's symptoms, medical history, and medical tests that let doctors look closely at the brain to see the type and location of the stroke.

There are many different ways to help people recover from a stroke. Drugs and physical therapy work to improve balance, coordination, and other deficits from the stroke such as speech and language problems. Occupational therapy can make it easier to do things like bathing and cooking. Many therapies start in the hospital and continue at home.

A family doctor can provide follow-up care. Progress is different for each person. Some people recover fully soon after a stroke. Others take months or even years. Sometimes the damage is so serious that therapy cannot help at all.

Lower Your Risk of Stroke

Talk to your doctor about what you can do to lower your risk of stroke. Even if you're in perfect health, follow these important suggestions:

- *Control your blood pressure.* Have your blood pressure checked often. If it is high, follow your doctor's advice to lower it. Treating high blood pressure lowers the risk of both stroke and heart disease.

- *Stop smoking.* Smoking is linked to increased risk for stroke. Quitting smoking at any age lowers the risk for stroke as well as for a lot of other serious diseases.

- *Exercise regularly.* Activities such as brisk walking, riding a bicycle, swimming, and yard work lower the risk of both stroke and heart disease. Researchers think that exercise may make the heart stronger and improve blood flow. Before you start a vigorous exercise program, be sure to check with your doctor.

- *Eat healthy foods.* Eat foods that are low in fats, cholesterol, and saturated fatty acids. Include a variety of fruits and vegetables in your daily diet.
- *Control your diabetes.* If you have diabetes, work with your doctor to get it under control. Untreated diabetes can damage blood vessels and lead to a build up of fatty deposits in the arteries (atherosclerosis). This narrows arteries and blocks normal blood flow. A blocked artery will lead to a stroke.

For More Information

Here are other resources for answers to your questions about stroke:

National Institute of Neurological Disorders and Stroke
Information Office
P.O. Box 5801
Bethesda, MD 20824-5801
800-352-9424 (toll-free)
www.ninds.nih.gov

National High Blood Pressure Education Program
NHLBI Health Information Center
P.O. Box 30105
Bethesda, MD 20824-0105
301-592-8573
www.nhlbi.nih.gov

National Stroke Association
9707 East Easter Lane
Englewood, CO 80112-3747
303-649-9299
800-787-6537 (toll-free)
www.stroke.org

American Stroke Association
7272 Greenville Avenue
Dallas, TX 75231
888-478-7653 (toll-free)
www.strokeassociation.org

For more information about health and aging, contact:

National Institute on Aging Information Center
P.O. Box 8057
Gaithersburg, MD 20898-8057
800-222-2225 (toll-free)
800-222-4225 (TTY/toll-free)

- To order publications (in English or Spanish) online, visit www.niapublications.org.
- The National Institute on Aging website is www.nia.nih.gov.
- Visit NIHSeniorHealth.gov (www.nihseniorhealth.gov), a senior-friendly website from the National Institute on Aging and the National Library of Medicine. This simple-to-use website features popular health topics for older adults. It has large type and a "talking" function that reads the text out loud.

July 2004

Urinary Incontinence

Are you reluctant to talk to your doctor about your bladder control problem? Don't be. There is help.

Loss of bladder control is called urinary incontinence. It can happen to anyone, but is very common in older people. At least one in ten people age 65 or older has this problem. Symptoms can range from mild leaking to uncontrollable wetting. Women are more likely than men to have incontinence.

Aging does not cause incontinence. It can occur for many reasons. For example, urinary tract infections, vaginal infection or irritation, constipation, and certain medicines can cause bladder control problems that last a short time. Sometimes incontinence lasts longer. This might be due to problems such as:

- Weak bladder muscles,
- Overactive bladder muscles,
- Blockage from an enlarged prostate,
- Damage to nerves that control the bladder from diseases such as multiple sclerosis or Parkinson's disease, or
- Diseases such as arthritis that can make walking painful and slow.

Many people with bladder control problems hide the problem from everyone, even from their doctor. There is no need to do that. **In most cases urinary incontinence can be treated and controlled, if not cured.** If you are having bladder control problems, don't suffer in silence. Talk to your doctor.

Bladder Control

The body stores urine in the bladder. During urination, muscles in the bladder contract or tighten. This forces urine out of the bladder and into a tube called the urethra that carries urine out of the body. At the same time, muscles surrounding the urethra relax and let the urine pass through. Spinal nerves control how these muscles move. Incontinence occurs if the bladder muscles contract or the muscles surrounding the urethra relax without warning.

Diagnosis

The first step in treating a bladder control problem is to see a doctor. He or she will give you a physical exam and take your medical history. The doctor will ask about your symptoms and the medicines you use. He or she will want to know if you have been sick recently or had surgery. Your doctor also may do a number of tests. These might include:

- Urine and blood tests, or
- Tests that measure how well you empty your bladder.

In addition, your doctor may ask you to keep a daily diary of when you urinate and when you leak urine. Your pattern of urinating and urine leakage may suggest which type of incontinence you have.

Types of Incontinence

There are several different types of urinary incontinence:

- *Stress incontinence* happens when urine leaks during exercise, coughing, sneezing, laughing, lifting heavy objects, or other body movements that put pressure on the bladder. It is the most common type of bladder control problem in younger and middle-age women. In some cases it is related to childbirth. It may also begin around the time of menopause.

- *Urge incontinence* happens when people can't hold their urine long enough to get to the toilet in time. Healthy people can have urge incontinence, but it is often found in people who have diabetes, stroke, Alzheimer's disease, Parkinson's disease, or multiple sclerosis. It is also sometimes an early sign of bladder cancer.

- *Overflow incontinence* happens when small amounts of urine leak from a bladder that is always full. A man can have trouble emptying his bladder if an enlarged prostate is blocking the urethra. Diabetes and spinal cord injury can also cause this type of incontinence.

- *Functional incontinence* happens in many older people who have normal bladder control. They just have a hard time getting to the toilet in time because of arthritis or other disorders that make moving quickly difficult.

Treatment

Today there are more treatments for urinary incontinence than ever before. The choice of treatment depends on the type of bladder control problem you have, how serious it is, and what best fits your lifestyle. As a general rule, the simplest and safest treatments should be tried first.

Bladder Control Training. Your doctor may suggest you try to get back control of your bladder through training. With bladder training you can change how your bladder stores and empties urine. There are several ways to do this:

- *Pelvic muscle exercises* (also known as Kegel exercises) work the muscles that you use to stop urinating. Making these muscles stronger helps you hold urine in your bladder longer. These exercises are easy to do. They can lessen or get rid of stress and urge incontinence.

- *Biofeedback* helps you become more aware of signals from your body. This may help you regain control over the muscles in your bladder and urethra. Biofeedback can be used to help teach pelvic muscle exercises.

- *Timed voiding* and *bladder training* also can help you control your bladder.

Kegel Exercises

The muscles you want to exercise are your pelvic floor muscles. These are the ones you use to stop the flow of urine or to keep from passing gas. Often doctors suggest that you squeeze and hold these muscles for a certain count, and then relax them. Then you repeat this a number of times. You will probably do this several times a day. Your doctor will give you exact directions.

In timed voiding, you keep a chart of urination and leaking to determine the pattern. Once you learn that, you can plan to empty your bladder before you might leak. When combined with biofeedback and pelvic muscle exercises, these methods may help you control urge and overflow incontinence.

Management

Besides bladder control training, there are several other ways to help manage incontinence:

- Sometimes doctors suggest a small, throwaway *patch*; a small, tampon-like *urethral plug*; or a vaginal insert called a *pessary* for women with stress incontinence.

- A doctor can prescribe *medicines* to treat incontinence. Some drugs prevent unwanted bladder contractions. Some relax muscles, helping the bladder to empty more fully during urination. Others tighten muscles in the bladder and urethra to cut down leakage. These drugs can sometimes cause side effects such as dry mouth, eye problems, or urine buildup. Vaginal estrogen may be helpful in women after menopause. Talk with your doctor about the benefits and side effects of using any of these medicines for a long time.

- A doctor can inject an *implant* into the area around the urethra. The implant adds bulk. This helps close the urethra to reduce stress incontinence. Injections may have to be repeated after a time because your body slowly gets rid of these substances.

- Sometimes *surgery* can improve or cure incontinence if it is caused by a problem such as a change in the position of the bladder or blockage due to an enlarged prostate. Common surgery for stress incontinence involves pulling the bladder up and securing it. When stress incontinence is serious, the surgeon may use a wide sling. This holds up the bladder and narrows the urethra to prevent leakage.

- You can now buy special absorbent *underclothing*. It is not bulky and can be worn easily under everyday clothing.

If you suffer from urinary incontinence, tell your doctor. Remember, under a doctor's care, incontinence can be treated and often cured. Even if treatment is not fully successful, careful managing can help you feel more relaxed and comfortable.

For More Information

You are not alone. There are people who can answer your questions and give you information about urinary incontinence. To learn more, contact:

National Association for Continence
P.O. Box 1019
Charleston, SC 29402-1019
800-252-3337 (toll-free)
www.nafc.org

Simon Foundation for Continence
P.O. Box 815
Wilmette, IL 60091
800-237-4666 (toll-free)
www.simonfoundation.org

National Institute of Diabetes and Digestive and Kidney Diseases
National Kidney and Urologic Diseases Information Clearinghouse
3 Information Way
Bethesda, MD 20892-3580
800-891-5390 (toll-free)
301-654-4415
www.niddk.nih.gov

For more information about health and aging, contact:

National Institute on Aging Information Center
P.O. Box 8057
Gaithersburg, MD 20898-8057
800-222-2225 (toll-free)
800-222-4225 (TTY/toll-free)

- To order publications (in English or Spanish) online, visit *www.niapublications.org*.
- The National Institute on Aging website is *www.nia.nih.gov*.
- Visit NIHSeniorHealth.gov (*www.nihseniorhealth.gov*), a senior-friendly website from the National Institute on Aging and the National Library of Medicine. This simple-to-use website features popular health topics for older adults. It has large type and a "talking" function that reads the text out loud.

August 2002

Staying Healthy
How to keep your body working well

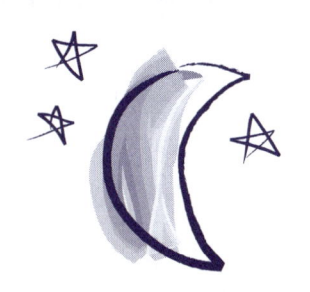

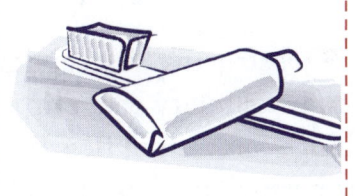

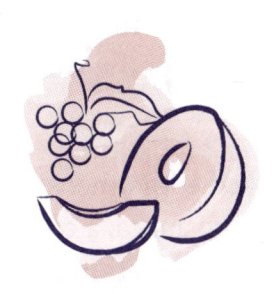

66	A Good Night's Sleep
69	Aging and Your Eyes
73	Alcohol Use and Abuse
76	Concerned About Constipation?
79	Dietary Supplements: More is Not Always Better
84	Exercise: Getting Fit for Life
88	Foot Care
91	Good Nutrition: It's a Way of Life
98	Life Extension: Science Fact or Science Fiction?
104	Sexuality in Later Life
109	Shots for Safety
114	Skin Care and Aging
120	Smoking: It's Never Too Late to Stop
125	Taking Care of Your Teeth and Mouth
129	What to Do About Flu

A Good Night's Sleep

We all look forward to a good night's sleep. Getting enough sleep and sleeping well help us stay healthy. Many older people do not enjoy a good night's sleep on a regular basis. They have trouble falling or staying asleep. Sleep patterns change as we age, but disturbed sleep and waking up tired every day is not part of normal aging. In fact, troubled sleep may be a sign of emotional or physical disorders and something you should talk about with a doctor or sleep specialist.

Sleep and Aging

There are two kinds of sleep in a normal sleep cycle—rapid eye movement or dreaming sleep (REM) and quiet sleep (non-REM). Everyone has about four or five cycles of REM and non-REM sleep a night. For older people, the amount of time spent in the deepest stages of non-REM sleep decreases. This may explain why older people are thought of as light sleepers.

Although the amount of sleep each person needs varies widely, the average range is between 7 and 8 hours a night. As we age, the amount of sleep we can expect to get at any one time drops off. By age 75, for many reasons, some people may find they are waking up several times each night. But, no matter what your age, talk to a doctor if your sleep patterns change.

Common Sleep Problems

At any age, insomnia is the most common sleep complaint. Insomnia means:

- Taking a long time to fall asleep (more than 30 to 45 minutes),
- Waking up many times each night,
- Waking up early and being unable to get back to sleep, or
- Waking up feeling tired.

With rare exceptions, insomnia is a symptom of a problem, not the problem itself.

Insomnia can be linked with other sleep disorders such as sleep apnea, a common problem that causes breathing to stop for periods of up to two minutes, many times each night. There are two kinds of sleep apnea:

- Obstructive sleep apnea is an involuntary pause in breathing—air cannot flow in or out of the person's nose or mouth.

- Central sleep apnea is less common and occurs when the brain doesn't send the right signals to start the breathing muscles.

In either case, the sleeper is totally unaware of his or her struggle to breathe.

Daytime sleepiness coupled with loud snoring at night are clues that you may have sleep apnea. A doctor specializing in sleep disorders can make a diagnosis and recommend treatment. Treatments include learning to sleep in the correct position, devices that help keep your airways open, medication, and surgery.

Suggestions for a Good Night's Sleep

A good night's sleep can make a big difference in how you feel. Here are some suggestions to help you:

- Follow a regular schedule—go to sleep and get up at the same time. Try not to nap too much during the day—you might be less sleepy at night.
- Try to exercise at regular times each day.
- Try to get some natural light in the afternoon each day.
- Be careful about what you eat. Don't drink beverages with caffeine late in the day. Caffeine is a stimulant and can keep you awake. Also, if you like a snack before bed, a warm beverage and a few crackers may help.
- Don't drink alcohol or smoke cigarettes to help you sleep. Even small amounts of alcohol can make it harder to stay asleep. Smoking is dangerous for many reasons including the hazard of falling asleep with a lit cigarette. The nicotine in cigarettes is also a stimulant.
- Create a safe and comfortable place to sleep. Make sure there are locks on all doors and smoke alarms on each floor. A lamp that's easy to turn on and a phone by your bed may be helpful. The room should be dark, well ventilated, and as quiet as possible.
- Develop a bedtime routine. Do the same things each night to tell your body that it's time to wind down. Some people watch the evening news, read a book, or soak in a warm bath.
- Use your bedroom only for sleeping. After turning off the light, give yourself about 15 minutes to fall asleep. If you are still awake and not drowsy, get out of bed. When you get sleepy, go back to bed.
- Try not to worry about your sleep. Some people find that playing mental games is helpful. For example, think black—a black cat on a black velvet pillow on a black corduroy sofa, etc.; or tell yourself it's five minutes before you have to get up and you're just trying to get a few extra winks.

If you are so tired during the day that you cannot function normally and if this lasts for more than 2–3 weeks, you should see your family doctor or a sleep disorders specialist.

For More Information

For general information about sleep, contact the following organizations:

American Sleep Apnea Association
1424 K Street, NW, Suite 302
Washington, DC 20005
202-293-3650
www.sleepapnea.org

Better Sleep Council
501 Wythe Street
Alexandria, VA 22314
703-683-8371
www.bettersleep.org

Narcolepsy Network
10921 Reed Hartman Highway
Suite 119
Cincinnati, Ohio 45242
513-891-3522
www.narcolepsynetwork.org

National Center for Sleep Disorders Research
Two Rockledge Center, Suite 10038
6701 Rockledge Drive, MSC 7920
Bethesda, MD 20892-7920
301-435-0199
www.nhlbi.nih.gov/health/public/sleep

National Sleep Foundation
1522 K Street, NW, Suite 500
Washington, DC 20005-1253
202-347-3471
www.sleepfoundation.org

Restless Legs Syndrome Foundation
819 Second Street, SW
Rochester, MN 55902
507-287-6465
www.rls.org/foundation

For more information about health and aging, contact:

National Institute on Aging Information Center
P.O. Box 8057
Gaithersburg, MD 20898-8057
800-222-2225 (toll-free)
800-222-4225 (TTY/toll-free)

- To order publications (in English or Spanish) online, visit *www.niapublications.org*.

- The National Institute on Aging website is *www.nia.nih.gov*.

- Visit NIHSeniorHealth.gov (*www.nihseniorhealth.gov*), a senior-friendly website from the National Institute on Aging and the National Library of Medicine. This simple-to-use website features popular health topics for older adults. It has large type and a "talking" function that reads the text out loud.

May 2000

Aging and Your Eyes

> Aunt Rose used to read all the time, but lately she complains that the words are blurry and hard to follow. Grandpa Joe just hammered his thumb for the third time this month. Last week Nancy's doctor suggested her mom needs cataract surgery.

Age can bring changes that affect your eyesight. But regular eye exams can help. With early detection, many eye problems can be treated and your risk of vision loss reduced.

Five Steps to Safeguard Your Eyesight

- Have regular physical exams by your doctor to check for diseases like diabetes. Such diseases can cause eye problems if not treated.
- Have a complete eye exam with an eye care professional every 1–2 years. The eye care professional should put drops in your eyes to enlarge (dilate) your pupils. This is the only way to find some eye diseases, such as glaucoma, that have no early signs or symptoms. The eye care professional should check your eyesight, your glasses, and your eye muscles.
- Find out if you are at high-risk for vision loss. Do you have a family history of diabetes or eye disease? If so, you need to have a dilated eye exam every year.
- See an eye care professional at once if you have any loss or dimness of eyesight, eye pain, fluid coming from the eye, double vision, redness, or swelling of your eye or eyelid.
- Wear sunglasses and a hat with a wide brim when outside. This will protect your eyes from too much sunlight, which can raise your risk of getting cataracts.

Common Eye Complaints

The following common eye complaints often happen with age. In most cases, they can be treated easily. Sometimes, they signal a more serious problem.

Presbyopia (prez-bee-OH-pee-uh) is a slow loss of ability to see close objects or small print. It is a normal process that happens as you get older. Signs of presbyopia include holding your reading materials at arm's length or getting headaches or tired eyes when you read or do other close work. Reading glasses can often fix the problem.

Floaters are tiny spots or specks that seem to float across your eyes. You might notice them in well-lit rooms or outdoors on a bright day. Floaters can be normal. But sometimes they are a sign of a more serious eye problem, such as retinal detachment. This often is the case if you

AGING AND YOUR EYES 69

see light flashes along with floaters. If you notice a sudden change in the type or number of spots or flashes, see your eye care professional right away.

Tearing (or having too many tears) can come from being sensitive to light, wind, or temperature changes. Tearing also can come from having dry eye. Protecting your eyes (by wearing sunglasses, for example) may solve the problem. Sometimes, tearing may mean a more serious eye problem, such as an infection or a blocked tear duct. Your eye care professional can treat both of these conditions.

Corneal diseases and conditions can cause redness, watery eyes, pain, reduced vision, or a halo effect. The cornea is the clear, dome-shaped "window" at the front of the eye. It helps to focus light that goes into the eye. Disease, infection, injury, toxic agents, and other things can harm the cornea. Treatments include changing your eyeglass prescription, using eye drops, or in severe cases, having surgery, including corneal transplantation. Corneal transplantation is a common treatment that works well and is safe.

Eyelid problems can come from different diseases or conditions. Common eyelid complaints include pain, itching, tearing, or being sensitive to light. Eyelid problems often can be treated with medicine or surgery.

Conjunctivitis (also called pink eye) happens when the tissue that lines the eyelids and covers the cornea becomes inflamed. It can cause itching, burning, tearing, or a feeling that something is in your eye. Conjunctivitis can be due to allergies or an infection. Infectious pinkeye can easily spread from one person to another. It is a common eye problem that your eye care professional can treat.

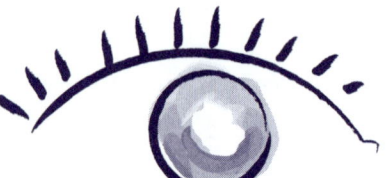

Eye Diseases and Disorders

The following eye problems are common with age. Often these can develop with few or no symptoms. Each can lead to vision loss and blindness. Having regular eye exams is the best way to protect yourself. If your eye care professional finds a problem early, a lot can be done to keep your eyesight.

Cataracts are cloudy areas in the eye's lens. Normal lenses are clear and let light through. Cataracts keep light from easily passing through the lens. This causes loss of eyesight. Cataracts often form slowly without any symptoms. Some stay small and don't change eyesight very much. Others may become large or thick and harm vision. Cataract surgery can help. Your eye care professional can watch for changes in your cataract over time to see if you need surgery. Cataract surgery is very safe. It is one of the most common surgeries done in the United States.

Dry eye happens when tear glands don't work well. Dry eye can be uncomfortable. It can cause itching, burning, or even some vision loss. Your eye care professional may suggest using a home humidifier or special eye drops (artificial tears). More serious cases of dry eye may need surgery.

Glaucoma comes from too much fluid pressure inside the eye. Over time, the disease can damage the optic nerve. This leads to vision loss and blindness. Loss of vision doesn't happen until there has been a large amount of nerve damage. Most people with glaucoma have no early symptoms or pain from increased pressure. You can protect yourself by having regular, dilated eye exams. Treatment may be prescription eye drops, medicines you take by mouth, or surgery.

Retinal disorders are a leading cause of blindness in the United States. The retina is a thin lining on the back of the eye. It is made up of cells that get visual images and pass them on to the brain. Retinal disorders that affect aging eyes include:

- *Age-related macular degeneration (AMD).* AMD affects the part of the retina (the macula) that gives you sharp central vision. Over time, AMD can ruin the sharp vision needed to see objects clearly and to do common tasks like driving and reading. In some cases, AMD can be treated with lasers to help reduce the risk of increased vision loss. Ask your eye care professional about recent research suggesting that some dietary supplements reduce the risk of AMD.
- *Diabetic retinopathy.* This common complication of diabetes happens when small blood vessels stop feeding the retina as they should. Laser surgery and a treatment called vitrectomy can help. If you have diabetes, be sure to have an eye exam through dilated pupils every year.
- *Retinal detachment.* This happens when the inner and outer layers of the retina become separated. If you notice changes in floaters and/or light flashes in your eye, either all at once or over time, see your eye care professional at once. With surgery or laser treatment, doctors often can reattach the retina and bring back all or part of your eyesight.

Low vision affects some people as they age. Low vision means you cannot fix your eyesight with glasses, contact lenses, medicine, or surgery. It can get in the way of your normal daily routine. You may have low vision if you:

- Have trouble seeing well enough to do everyday tasks like reading, cooking, or sewing,
- Can't recognize the faces of friends or family,
- Have trouble reading street signs, or
- Find that lights don't seem as bright as usual.

If you have any of these problems, ask your eye care professional to test you for low vision. There are many things that can help. Aids can help you read, write, and manage daily living tasks. Lighting can be adjusted to your needs. You also can try prescription reading glasses, large-print reading materials, magnifying aids, closed-circuit televisions, audio tapes, electronic reading machines, and computers that use large print and speech.

Other simple changes also may help:

- Write with bold, black felt-tip markers.
- Use paper with bold lines to help you write in a straight line.
- Put colored tape on the edge of your steps to help you avoid a fall.
- Install dark-colored light switches and electrical outlets that you can see easily against light-colored walls.
- Use motion lights that turn on by themselves when you enter a room.

These may help you avoid accidents caused by poor lighting.

- Use telephones, clocks, and watches with large numbers, and put large-print labels on the microwave and stove.

Less than perfect vision does not have to hamper your lifestyle. By having regular eye exams you will be doing your part to take care of your eyes.

For More Information   To learn more about eye care contact:

The National Eye Institute (NEI)
2020 Vision Place
Bethesda, MD 20892-3655
301-496-5248
www.nei.nih.gov

For more information about health and aging, contact:

National Institute on Aging Information Center
P.O. Box 8057
Gaithersburg, MD 20898-8057
800-222-2225 (toll-free)
800-222-4225 (TTY/toll-free)

- To order publications (in English or Spanish) online, visit *www.niapublications.org*.
- The National Institute on Aging website is *www.nia.nih.gov*.

- Visit NIHSeniorHealth.gov (*www.nihseniorhealth.gov*), a senior-friendly website from the National Institute on Aging and the National Library of Medicine. This simple-to-use website features popular health topics for older adults. It has large type and a "talking" function that reads the text out loud.

September 2002

Alcohol Use and Abuse

Anyone at any age can have a drinking problem. Great-Uncle George may have always liked his liquor, so his family may not see that his drinking behavior is getting worse as he gets older. Grandma Betty was a teetotaler all her life—she started having a drink each night to help her get to sleep after her husband died. Now no one realizes that she needs a couple of drinks to get through each day.

These are common stories. The fact is that families, friends, and health care professionals often overlook their concerns about older people's drinking. Sometimes trouble with alcohol in older people is mistaken for other conditions that happen with age. But alcohol use deserves special attention. Because the aging process affects how the body handles alcohol, the same amount of alcohol can have a greater effect as a person grows older. Over time, someone whose drinking habits haven't changed may find she or he has a problem.

Facts About Alcohol and Aging

- Some research has shown that as people age they become more sensitive to alcohol's effects. In other words, the same amount of alcohol can have a greater effect on an older person than on someone who is younger.
- Some medical risks, such as high blood pressure, ulcers, and diabetes, can worsen with alcohol use.
- Many medicines—both prescription and over-the-counter—can be dangerous or even deadly when mixed with alcohol. This is a special worry for older people because the average person over age 65 takes at least two medicines a day. Here are some examples: aspirin can cause bleeding in the stomach and intestines. If you take aspirin while drinking alcohol, the risk of bleeding is much higher. Cold and allergy medicines (antihistamines) often make people sleepy. When alcohol is combined with those medicines, it can make drowsiness worse and driving even more dangerous. Alcohol used with large doses of the pain killer acetaminophen can raise the risk of liver damage. If you are taking any over-the-counter or prescription medications, ask your doctor or pharmacist if you can safely drink alcohol.

Effects of Alcohol

Even drinking a small amount of alcohol can impair judgment, coordination, and reaction time. It can increase the risk of work and household accidents, including falls and hip fractures. It also adds to the risk of car crashes—a special concern because almost 10 percent of this nation's drivers are over age 65.

Heavy drinking over time also can cause certain cancers, liver cirrhosis, immune system disorders, and brain damage.

Alcohol can make some medical concerns hard for doctors to find and treat. For example, alcohol causes changes in the heart and blood vessels. These changes can dull pain that might be a warning sign of a heart attack. Drinking also can make older people forgetful and confused. These symptoms could be mistaken for signs of Alzheimer's disease. For people with diabetes, drinking affects blood sugar levels. Ulcers also may become worse with alcohol use.

> **The National Institute on Alcohol Abuse and Alcoholism, part of the National Institutes of Health, recommends that people over age 65 who choose to drink have no more than one drink a day. Drinking at this level usually is not associated with health risks.**

People who drink more than a little alcohol also may be putting themselves at risk for serious conflicts with family, friends, and coworkers. The more heavily they drink, the greater the chance for trouble at home, at work, with friends, and even with strangers.

How to Know if Someone Has a Drinking Problem

There are two types of problem drinkers: early and late onset. Some people have been heavy drinkers for many years. But, as with Great-Uncle George, over time the same amount of liquor packs a more powerful punch. Other people, like Grandma Betty, develop a drinking problem later in life. Sometimes this is due to major life changes like shifts in employment, failing health, or the death of friends or loved ones. Often these life changes can bring loneliness, boredom, anxiety, and depression. In fact, depression in older adults often goes along with alcohol misuse. At first, a drink seems to bring relief from stressful situations. Later on, drinking can start to cause trouble.

Not everyone who drinks regularly has a drinking problem, and not all problem drinkers drink every day. You might want to get help if you or a loved one:

- Drink to calm your nerves, forget your worries, or reduce depression,
- Lose interest in food,
- Gulp down drinks,
- Frequently have more than three drinks in one day (a standard drink is one 12-ounce bottle or can of beer or a wine cooler, one 5-ounce glass of wine, or 1.5 ounces of 80-proof distilled spirits),
- Lie about or try to hide drinking habits,
- Drink alone,
- Hurt yourself, or someone else, while drinking,
- Were drunk more than three or four times last year,
- Need more alcohol to get high,
- Feel irritable, resentful, or unreasonable when not drinking, or
- Have medical, social, or financial worries caused by drinking.

Getting Help

Studies show that older problem drinkers are as able to benefit from treatment as are younger alcohol abusers. To get help, talk to your doctor. He or she can give you advice about your health, drinking, and treatment options. Your local health department or social services agencies can also help.

There are many types of treatments available. Some, such as 12-step help programs, have been around a long time. Others include getting alcohol out of the body (detoxification), taking prescription medicines to help prevent a return to drinking once you have stopped, and individual and/or group counseling. Newer programs teach people with drinking problems to learn which situations or feelings trigger the urge to drink as well as ways to cope without alcohol. Because the support of family members is important, many programs also counsel married couples and family members as part of the treatment process. Programs may also link individuals with important community resources.

Scientists continue to study alcohol's effects on people and to look for new ways to treat alcoholism. This research

For More Information

Contact these groups to learn more about alcohol abuse:

National Institute on Alcohol Abuse and Alcoholism (NIAAA)
5635 Fishers Lane, MSC 9304
Bethesda, MD 20892-9304
301-443-3860
www.niaaa.nih.gov

National Drug and Treatment Referral Routing Service
National Clearinghouse for Alcohol and Drug Information
Substance Abuse and Mental Health Services Administration
800-729-6686 (toll-free)
www.health.org

Alcoholics Anonymous (AA)
Grand Central Station
P.O. Box 459
New York, NY 10163
212-870-3400
www.aa.org

National Council on Alcoholism and Drug Dependence, Inc. (NCADD)
22 Cortlandt Street, Suite 801
New York, NY 10007
www.ncadd.org

- Hope Line: 800-622-2255 (toll-free)

For more information about health and aging, contact:

National Institute on Aging Information Center
P.O. Box 8057
Gaithersburg, MD 20898-8057
800-222-2225 (toll-free)
800-222-4225 (TTY/toll-free)

- To order publications (in English or Spanish) online, visit www.niapublications.org.
- The National Institute on Aging website is www.nia.nih.gov.

- Visit NIHSeniorHealth.gov (www.nihseniorhealth.gov), a senior-friendly website from the National Institute on Aging and the National Library of Medicine. This simple-to-use website features popular health topics for older adults. It has large type and a "talking" function that reads the text out loud.

September 2002

Concerned About Constipation?

Nearly everyone becomes constipated at one time or another. Usually, it is not serious. To avoid most constipation problems, it helps to know what causes it, how to prevent it, and how to treat it.

Constipation is a symptom, not a disease. You may be constipated if you are having fewer bowel movements than usual, with a long or hard passing of stools. Older people are more likely than younger people to become constipated.

Experts agree that older people often worry too much about having a bowel movement every day. There is no right number of daily or weekly bowel movements. Being regular is different for each person. For some people, it can mean bowel movements twice a day. For others, movements just twice a week are normal.

Questions to Ask

Some doctors suggest asking these questions to decide if you are constipated:

- Do you often have fewer than three bowel movements each week?
- Do you often have a hard time passing stools?
- Is there pain?
- Are there other problems such as bleeding?

Did you answer "yes" to more than one of these questions? If so, you may have a constipation problem. Otherwise, you probably do not.

What Causes Constipation?

Doctors do not always know what causes constipation. Eating a poor diet, not drinking enough water, or using laxatives too often can be causes. Also, some medicines can lead to constipation. These include some antidepressants, antacids containing aluminum or calcium, antihistamines, diuretics, and antiparkinsonism drugs.

The role of diet. People may become constipated if they do not eat enough high-fiber foods like vegetables, fruits, and whole grains. Some research shows that high-fiber diets can help prevent constipation. Eating a lot of high-fat meats, dairy products and eggs, or rich desserts and sugary sweets also may cause constipation.

People who live alone sometimes lose interest in cooking and eating. As a result, they start using a lot of prepared foods.

These foods tend to be low in fiber and so may lead to constipation. In addition, bad teeth can cause older people to choose soft, processed foods that contain small amounts of fiber.

People sometimes do not drink enough fluids. This often is true when people are not eating regular meals. But water and other liquids are important. They add bulk to stools, which helps make bowel movements easier.

Misuse of laxatives and enemas. Many people think of laxatives as a cure for constipation. But heavy use of laxatives often is not needed, and laxatives can become habit forming. If you use laxatives too often, your body can begin to rely on them to bring on bowel movements. (Using laxatives too often also can cause diarrhea.) Over time, your body will forget how to work on its own.

For the same reason, if you use enemas too often, your body may begin to depend on them. Too many enemas may stop you from having normal bowel movements. Too much mineral oil, another popular laxative, can lower your body's ability to use key vitamins (A, D, E, and K). Sometimes mineral oil, if taken along with other drugs that stop blood clots (anticoagulants), can cause unwanted side effects.

Other causes of constipation. Lack of exercise or long periods in bed, such as after an accident or illness, may cause constipation. Doctors sometimes suggest medicine for people who stay in bed and suffer from chronic constipation. But being more active, when possible, is best.

People also can become constipated if they ignore their natural urge to have a bowel movement. Some people prefer to have bowel movements only at home. But holding in a bowel movement can cause constipation if the delay is too long.

In some people, disorders or a blockage of the intestines may cause constipation. These disorders may affect the muscles or nerves responsible for normal bowel movements. A doctor can perform tests to see if a problem like this is the cause of constipation. If so, the problem often can be treated.

Treatment

If you become constipated, first see your doctor to rule out a more serious problem. If test results show no disease or blockage, and if your doctor approves, try these remedies:

- Increase fiber by eating more fresh fruits and vegetables, either cooked or raw, and more whole-grain cereals and breads. Dried fruit such as apricots, prunes, and figs are especially high in fiber.

- Drink plenty of liquids (1–2 quarts daily), unless you have heart, blood vessel, or kidney problems. (But keep in mind that some people can become constipated from drinking large amounts of milk.)

- Some doctors suggest adding small amounts of unprocessed bran ("miller's bran") to baked goods, cereals, and fruit. Some people suffer from bloating and gas for several weeks after adding bran to their diets. Make diet changes slowly to allow your digestive system to adapt. Remember, if your diet is well balanced and contains a variety of foods high in natural fiber, it may not be necessary to add bran to other foods.
- Stay active.

Do not expect to have a bowel movement every day or even every other day. Remember, being regular is different for each person. If your bowel movements are usually painless and occur regularly (whether 2 times a day or 3 times a week), you are probably not constipated.

If you still have concerns about constipation, check with your doctor to find out what you should do.

For More Information

You can get more information about constipation from:

National Institute of Diabetes and Digestive and Kidney Diseases
National Digestive Diseases Information Clearinghouse
2 Information Way
Bethesda, MD 20892-3570
800-891-5389 (toll-free)
301-654-3810
www.niddk.nih.gov

For more information about health and aging, contact:

National Institute on Aging Information Center
P.O. Box 8057
Gaithersburg, MD 20898-8057
800-222-2225 (toll-free)
800-222-4225 (TTY/toll-free)

- To order publications (in English or Spanish) online, visit www.niapublications.org.
- The National Institute on Aging website is www.nia.nih.gov.

- Visit NIHSeniorHealth.gov (www.nihseniorhealth.gov), a senior-friendly website from the National Institute on Aging and the National Library of Medicine. This simple-to-use website features popular health topics for older adults. It has large type and a "talking" function that reads the text out loud.

January 2002

Dietary Supplements: More is Not Always Better

> Bill's retired and lives alone. Often he's just not hungry or is too tired to fix a whole meal. Does he need a multi-vitamin or one of those dietary supplements he sees in ads everywhere? He wonders if they work—will one help his arthritis, or another give him more energy? And, are they safe?

"Dietary supplements" used to make you think only of vitamins and minerals. But, today this big business makes and sells many different types of dietary supplements that have vitamins, minerals, fiber, amino acids, herbs, or hormones in them. Supplements come in the form of pills, capsules, powders, gel tabs, extracts, or liquids. Sometimes you find them added to drinks or energy bars. They might be used to add nutrients to your diet or to prevent health problems. You don't even need a prescription from your doctor to buy dietary supplements.

Do I Need a Dietary Supplement?

Ads for supplements seem to promise to make you feel better, keep you from getting sick, or even help you live longer. Often there is little, if any, scientific support for these claims. In fact, some supplements can hurt you. Others are a waste of money because they don't give you any health benefits.

So, should you take a supplement? You might want to talk to your doctor or a registered dietitian to answer that question. A friend or neighbor, or someone on a commercial, shouldn't be suggesting a supplement for you.

Are These Supplements Safe?

Are you thinking about using dietary supplements? Remember that these "over-the-counter" substances are not like the penicillin or blood pressure medicine your doctor might prescribe for you. The U.S. Food and Drug Administration (FDA) has to check prescription drugs to make sure they are safe and do what they promise before they are sold. The same is true for "over-the-counter drugs" like cold and pain medicines. It is not the FDA's job to check dietary supplements in the same way. That means they are not reviewed by the FDA before being sold, but it is the FDA's job to take action against unsafe products on the market. Only if enough people report problems with a dietary supplement, can the FDA study these possible problems and take action.

Besides the FDA, many federal government agencies and private groups are interested in dietary supplements. The National Institutes of Health (NIH) is the Federal focal point for medical research in the United States. NIH supports research studies looking at the safety and helpfulness of some of the ingredients found in many supplements.

Business and consumer groups are also interested in dietary supplements. So are private professional groups such as the National Academy of Sciences (NAS). The NAS develops guidelines saying how much of each vitamin and mineral people need.

What About Vitamins and Minerals?

Vitamins and minerals are nutrients found naturally in food. We need them to stay healthy. The benefits and side effects of many vitamins and minerals have been studied. *The best way to get vitamins and minerals is through the food you eat, not any supplements you might take.* Try to eat the number of servings of food recommended by the U.S. Department of Agriculture's Food Guide Pyramid each day (see chart). Pick foods that are lower in fat and added sugars. If you can't eat enough, then ask your doctor if you should be taking a multivitamin and mineral supplement. And remember:

- The supplement doesn't need to be a "senior" formula.
- It shouldn't have large or "mega-doses" of vitamins and minerals.
- Generally store or generic brands are fine.

How much should you take? The NAS has developed recommendations for vitamins and minerals. Check the label on your supplement bottle. It shows the level of vitamins and minerals in a serving compared with the suggested daily intake.

How Many Servings Do You Need?

Bread, cereal, rice, and pasta: *5-10 servings,*

Vegetables: *2-3½ cups,*

Fruits: *1½ -2½ cups,*

Milk, yogurt, and cheese: *3 servings,*

Meat, poultry, fish, dry beans, eggs, and nuts: *2–3 servings,*

Fats, oils, and sweets: *use sparingly.*

For example, a vitamin A intake of 100 percent DV (Daily Value) means the supplement is giving you the full amount of vitamin A you need each day. This is *in addition* to what you are getting from your food.

Some people might think that if a little is good, a lot must be better. But, that doesn't necessarily apply to vitamins and minerals. Depending on the supplement, your age, and your health, taking more than 100 percent DV could be harmful to your health. Also, if your body cannot use the entire supplement you take, you've wasted money. Finally, large doses of some vitamins and minerals can also keep your prescription medications from working as they should.

Anything Special for People Over 50?

Even if you eat a good variety of foods, if you are over 50, you might need certain supplements. Talk to your doctor or a registered dietitian. Depending on your needs, he or she might suggest you get the following amounts from food and, if needed, supplements:

- *Vitamin B_{12}*—2.4 mcg (micrograms) of B_{12} each day. Some foods, such as cereals, are fortified with this vitamin. But, up to one-third of older people can no longer absorb natural vitamin B_{12} from their food. They need this vitamin to keep their blood and nerves healthy.
- *Calcium*—1,200 mg (milligrams), but not more than 2,500 mg a day. As you age, you need more of this and vitamin D to keep bones strong and to keep the bone you have. Bone loss can lead to fractures, mainly of the hip, spine, or wrist, in both older women and men.
- *Vitamin D*—400 IU (international units) for people age 51 to 70 and 600 IU for those over 70, but not more than 2,000 IU each day.
- *Iron*—extra iron for women past menopause who are using menopausal hormone therapy (men and other postmenopausal women need 8 mg of iron). Iron helps keep red blood cells healthy. Postmenopausal women who use menopausal hormone therapy may still experience a monthly period. They need extra iron to make up for that loss of blood.
- *Vitamin B_6*—1.7 mg for men and 1.5 mg for women. This vitamin is needed for forming red blood cells and to keep you healthy.

Sources of Calcium

- **Dairy products like milk and cheese and foods made with them,**
- **Canned fish with soft bones like salmon and sardines,**
- **Dark green leafy vegetables,**
- **Calcium-fortified products such as orange juice, and**
- **Breads and cereals made with calcium-fortified flour.**

Non-dairy calcium sources are especially good for people who cannot use dairy products.

What Are Antioxidants?

You may have heard about the possible benefits of *antioxidants*, natural substances found in food. Right now, there is no proof that large doses of antioxidants will prevent chronic diseases such as heart disease, diabetes, or cataracts. Eating fruits and vegetables (at least five servings a day) rather than taking a supplement is the best way to get antioxidants. Vegetable oil and nuts are also good sources of some antioxidants.

What About Herbal Supplements?

You may have heard of ginkgo biloba, ginseng, Echinacea, or black cohosh. These are examples of herbal supplements. They are dietary supplements that come from certain plants. It's easy to think they are safe because they come from plants. And, although herbal supplements are not approved as drugs, some are being studied as possible treatments for illness. But, it's still too soon to tell. Remember some strong poisons like hemlock and prescription medicines such as cancer drugs come from plants as well. You need to be careful.

When you use any dietary supplement, including herbals, for a health problem, you are using that supplement as a drug. Because their ingredients may have an effect on your body, they can interfere with medications you may already be taking. Some herbal supplements can also cause serious side effects such as high blood pressure, nausea, diarrhea, constipation, fainting, headaches, seizures, heart attack, or stroke.

What's Best for Me?

If you are thinking about using dietary supplements for any reason, remember:

- Talk to your doctor or a registered dietitian. Just because something worked for your neighbor, doesn't mean the same will be true for you.
- Use only the supplement your doctor or dietitian and you decide on—don't buy combinations that have things you don't want or need.
- If your doctor does not suggest a dietary supplement, but you decide to use one anyway, tell your doctor. Then he or she can keep an eye on your health and adjust your other medications if needed.
- Learn as much as you can about the supplement you are thinking about, but be aware of the source of the information. Could the writer or group profit from the sale of a particular supplement?
- Buy brands you know from companies you, your doctor, your dietitian, or your pharmacist know are reputable.
- Remember that many of the claims made about supplements are not based on enough scientific proof. If you have questions about a supplement, contact the firm and ask if it has information on the safety and/or effectiveness of the ingredients in its product.

What Else Can I Do?

Here's what one active older person does:

When Pearl was nearing 60, she was concerned about remaining healthy and

82 BOUND FOR YOUR GOOD HEALTH: A COLLECTION OF AGE PAGES *active as she aged. She began to exercise. Now she takes a long, brisk walk 3 to 4 times a week. In bad weather, she joins the mall walkers at the local shopping mall. In good weather, she also works in her garden. She has long since stopped smoking. Pearl tries to follow a healthy diet. She reads the newspaper everyday. She's even learning how to use a computer and keeps in touch with her family by e-mail, as well as phone calls. She always wears a seatbelt when in a car. Last month, she danced at her granddaughter's wedding. Pearl is now 84 years old.*

Try following Pearl's example—stick to a healthy diet, exercise, keep your mind active, don't smoke, and see your doctor regularly.

For More Information

The following are some resources for information on vitamins, minerals, other dietary supplements, and nutrition:

Center for Food Safety and Applied Nutrition
Food and Drug Administration
5100 Paint Branch Parkway
College Park, MD 20740-3835
888-723-3366 (toll-free)
www.cfsan.fda.gov

Food and Nutrition Information Center
Department of Agriculture
10301 Baltimore Avenue
Room 105
Beltsville, MD 20705-2351
301-504-5719
www.nal.usda.gov/fnic

Office of Dietary Supplements
National Institutes of Health
6100 Executive Boulevard
Room 3B01, MSC 7517
Bethesda, MD 20892-7517
301-435-2920
http://dietary-supplements.info.nih.gov

For more information about health and aging, contact:

National Institute on Aging Information Center
P.O. Box 8057
Gaithersburg, MD 20898-8057
800-222-2225 (toll-free)
800-222-4225 (TTY/toll-free)

- To order publications (in English or Spanish) online, visit www.niapublications.org.
- The National Institute on Aging website is www.nia.nih.gov.

- Visit NIHSeniorHealth.gov (*www.nihseniorhealth.gov*), a senior-friendly website from the National Institute on Aging and the National Library of Medicine. This simple-to-use website features popular health topics for older adults. It has large type and a "talking" function that reads the text out loud.

August 2002

Exercise: Getting Fit For Life

> "I don't have time."
>
> "I'm too old—I might hurt myself."
>
> "I'd be too embarrassed at a gym with all those fit young people around."

Sound familiar? Maybe one of these is the reason you aren't physically active or exercising. But, in fact, scientists now know that it's usually more dangerous to not exercise, no matter how old you are. And you don't need to buy fancy clothes or belong to a gym to become more active.

Most older people don't get enough physical activity. Here are some reasons why they should:

- Lack of physical activity and not eating the right foods, taken together, are the second greatest underlying cause of death in the United States. (Smoking is the number one cause.)
- Exercise can help older people feel better and enjoy life more. No one is too old or too out of shape to be more active.
- Regular exercise can prevent or delay some diseases like cancer, heart disease, or diabetes. It can also perk up your mood and help depression, too.
- Being active can help older people to stay independent and able to keep doing things like getting around or dressing themselves.

So, make physical activity a part of your everyday life. Find things you enjoy. Go for brisk walks. Ride a bike. Dance. Work around the house and in the yard. Take care of your garden. Climb stairs. Rake leaves. Do a mix of things that keep you moving and active.

Four Types of Exercise

There are four types of exercises you need to do to have the right mixture of physical activities.

1. Be sure to get at least 30 minutes of activity that makes you breathe harder on most or all days of the week. That's called "endurance activity," because it builds your energy or "staying power." You don't have to be active for 30 minutes all at once. Ten minutes of endurance activity at a time is fine. Just make sure those 10-minute sessions add up to a total of 30 minutes most days.

How hard do you need to push yourself? One doctor describes the right level of effort this way: If you can talk without any trouble at all, you're not working hard enough. If you can't talk at all, it's too hard.

2. Keep using your muscles. When muscles aren't used, they waste away at any age.

How important is it to have "enough" muscle? Very! When you have enough muscle, you can get up from a chair by yourself. When you don't—you have to wait for someone to help you. When you have enough muscle, you can walk through the park with your grandchildren. When you don't, you have to stay home. That's true for younger adults as well as for people age 90 and older.

Keeping your muscles in shape can help prevent another serious problem in older people—falls that cause problems like broken hips. When the leg and hip muscles that support you are strong, you're less likely to fall. Even if you do fall, you will be more likely to be able to get up on your own. And using your muscles may make your bones stronger, too.

3. Do things to help your balance. For example, stand on one foot, then the other. If you can, don't hold on to anything for support. Stand up from sitting in a chair without using your hands or arms. Every now and then walk heel-to-toe. When you walk this way, the toes of the foot in back should almost touch the heel of the foot in front.

4. Stretch. Stretching can help keep you flexible. You will be able to move more freely. Stretch when your muscles are warmed up. Never stretch so far that it hurts.

Who Should Exercise?

Almost anyone, at any age, can improve his or her health by doing some type of activity. But, check with your doctor first if you plan to do strenuous activity (the kind that makes you breathe hard and sweat) and you are a man over 40 or a woman over 50. Your doctor might be able to give you a go-ahead over the phone, or he or she might ask you to come in for a visit.

You can still exercise even if you have a long-term condition like heart disease or diabetes. In fact, physical activity may help your illness, but only if it's done during times when your condition is under control. During flare-ups, exercise could be harmful. If you have any of the following problems, it's important to check with your doctor before starting an exercise program:

- A chronic disease, or a high risk of getting one—for example, if you smoke, if you are obese, or if you have a family history of a long-term disease,
- Any new symptom you haven't talked about with your doctor,
- Chest pain,
- Shortness of breath,
- The feeling that your heart is skipping, racing, or fluttering,
- Blood clots,
- Infections or fever,
- Unplanned weight loss,
- Foot or ankle sores that won't heal,
- Joint swelling,
- Pain or trouble walking after you've fallen,
- A bleeding or detached retina, eye surgery, or laser treatment,
- A hernia, or
- Hip surgery.

EXERCISE: GETTING FIT FOR LIFE 85

Safety Tips

Here are some things you can do to make sure you are exercising safely:

- Start slowly. Little by little build up your activities and how hard you work at them. Doing too much, too soon, can hurt you, especially if you have not been active.

- Don't hold your breath while straining—when using your muscles, for example. That could cause changes in your blood pressure. It may seem strange at first, but the rule is to breathe out while your muscle is working, breathe in when it relaxes. For example, if you are lifting something, breathe out as you lift; breathe in when you stop.

- If you are taking any medicines or have any illnesses that change your natural heart rate, don't use your pulse rate as a way of judging how hard you should exercise. One example of this kind of medicine is a type of blood pressure drug known as a beta blocker.

- Use safety equipment to keep you from getting hurt. That means, for example, a helmet for bike riding or the right shoes for walking or jogging.

- Unless your doctor has asked you to limit fluids, be sure to drink plenty when you are doing activities that make you sweat. Many older people tend to be low on fluid much of the time, even when not exercising.

- Always bend forward from the hips, not the waist. If you keep your back straight, you're probably bending the right way. If your back "humps," that's probably wrong.

- Warm up your muscles before you stretch. For example, do a little easy biking, or walking and light arm pumping first.

Exercises should not hurt or make you feel really tired. You might feel some soreness, a little discomfort, or a bit weary, but you should not feel pain. In fact, in many ways, being physically active will probably make you feel better.

How to Find Out More

Local gyms, universities, or hospitals might be able to help you find a teacher or program that works for you. You can also check with nearby churches or synagogues, senior and civic centers, parks, recreation associations, YMCAs, YWCAs, or even area shopping malls for exercise, wellness, or walking programs.

Looking for a safe exercise program? The National Institute on Aging (NIA) publishes *Exercise: A Guide from the National Institute on Aging*. This free 80-page booklet has instructions and drawings for many strength, balance, and stretching exercises you can do at home. Will they work? Scientific research supported by the NIA helped experts develop these exercises so they should help you if you do them as described. You can get the guide in English or Spanish. In addition, the NIA has a 48-minute exercise video for $7. You can order the video from the NIA Information Center.

For More Information

Many organizations have information for older people about physical activity and exercise. The following list will help you get started:

American College of Sports Medicine
P.O. Box 1440
Indianapolis, IN 46206-1440
317-637-9200
www.acsm.org

American Physical Therapy Association
1111 North Fairfax Street
Alexandria, VA 22314-1488
800-999-2782 (toll-free)
www.apta.org

Centers for Disease Control and Prevention
1600 Clifton Road
Atlanta, GA 30333
800-311-3435 (toll-free)
www.cdc.gov

Fifty-Plus Lifelong Fitness
2483 East Bayshore Road
Suite 202
Palo Alto, CA 94303
650-843-1750
www.50plus.org

National Library of Medicine MedlinePlus
www.medlineplus.gov

- In Health Topics, go to: "Exercise for Seniors"

The President's Council on Physical Fitness and Sports
200 Independence Avenue, SW
Room 738-H, Department W
Washington, DC 20201-0004
202-690-9000
http://fitness.gov

Small Steps
www.smallstep.gov

For more information about health and aging, contact:

National Institute on Aging Information Center
P.O. Box 8057
Gaithersburg, MD 20898-8057
800-222-2225 (toll-free)
800-222-4225 (TTY/toll-free)

- To order publications (in English or Spanish) online, visit *www.niapublications.org*.

- The National Institute on Aging website is *www.nia.nih.gov*.

- Visit NIHSeniorHealth.gov (*www.nihseniorhealth.gov*), a senior-friendly website from the National Institute on Aging and the National Library of Medicine. This simple-to-use website features popular health topics for older adults. It has large type and a "talking" function that reads the text out loud.

May 2004

EXERCISE: GETTING FIT FOR LIFE

Foot Care

> When we are in love, we may be "swept off our feet." When we don't want to do something, we are said to have "cold feet." A sensible person "has both feet on the ground." Sometimes we even "vote with our feet."

Years of wear and tear can be hard on our feet. So can disease, poor circulation, improperly trimmed toenails, and wearing shoes that don't fit properly. Problems with our feet can be the first sign of more serious medical conditions such as arthritis, diabetes, and nerve and circulatory disorders.

Preventing Foot Trouble

Practice good foot care. Check your feet regularly, or have a member of your family check them. Podiatrists and primary care doctors (internists and family practitioners) are qualified to treat most foot problems. Sometimes the special skills of an orthopedic surgeon or dermatologist are needed.

It also helps to keep blood circulating to your feet as much as possible. Do this by putting your feet up when you are sitting or lying down, stretching if you've had to sit for a long while, walking, having a gentle foot massage, or taking a warm foot bath. Try to avoid pressure from shoes that don't fit right. Try not to expose your feet to cold temperatures. Don't sit for long periods of time (especially with your legs crossed). Don't smoke.

Wearing comfortable shoes that fit well can prevent many foot ailments. Here are some tips for getting a proper shoe fit:

- The size of your feet changes as you grow older so always have your feet measured before buying shoes. The best time to measure your feet is at the end of the day when your feet are largest.
- Most of us have one foot that is larger than the other, so fit your shoe to your larger foot.
- Don't select shoes by the size marked inside the shoe but by how the shoe fits your foot.
- Select a shoe that is shaped like your foot.
- During the fitting process, make sure there is enough space (3/8" to 1/2") for your longest toe at the end of each shoe when you are standing up.
- Make sure the ball of your foot fits comfortably into the widest part of the shoe.
- Don't buy shoes that feel too tight and expect them to stretch to fit.
- Your heel should fit comfortably in the shoe with a minimum amount of slipping—the shoes should not ride up and down on your heel when you walk.

- Walk in the shoes to make sure they fit and feel right. Then take them home and spend some time walking on carpet to make sure the fit is a good one.

The upper part of the shoes should be made of a soft, flexible material to match the shape of your foot. Shoes made of leather can reduce the possibility of skin irritations. Soles should provide solid footing and not be slippery. Thick soles cushion your feet when walking on hard surfaces. Low-heeled shoes are more comfortable, safer, and less damaging than high-heeled shoes.

Common Foot Problems

Fungal and bacterial conditions, including athlete's foot, occur because our feet spend a lot of time in shoes—a warm, dark, humid place that is perfect for fungi to grow. Fungal and bacterial conditions can cause dry skin, redness, blisters, itching, and peeling. If not treated right away, an infection may be hard to cure. If not treated properly, the infection may reoccur. To prevent infections, keep your feet—especially the area between your toes—clean and dry. Change your shoes and socks or stockings often to help keep your feet dry. Try dusting your feet daily with foot powder. If your foot condition does not get better within 2 weeks, talk to your doctor.

Dry skin can cause itching and burning feet. Use mild soap in small amounts and a moisturizing cream or lotion on your legs and feet every day. Be careful about adding oils to bath water since they can make your feet and bathtub very slippery.

Corns and calluses are caused by friction and pressure when the bony parts of your feet rub against your shoes. If you have corns or calluses, see your doctor. Sometimes wearing shoes that fit better or using special pads solves the problem. Treating corns and calluses yourself may be harmful, especially if you have diabetes or poor circulation. Over-the-counter medicines contain acids that destroy the tissue but do not treat the cause. Sometimes these medicines reduce the need for surgery, but check with your doctor before using them.

Warts are skin growths caused by viruses. They are sometimes painful and, if untreated, may spread. Since over-the-counter preparations rarely cure warts, see your doctor. A doctor can apply medicines, burn or freeze the wart off, or take the wart off with surgery.

Bunions develop when the joints in your big toe no longer fit together as they should and become swollen and tender. Bunions tend to run in families. If a bunion is not severe, wearing shoes cut wide at the instep and toes, taping the foot, or wearing pads that cushion the bunion may help the pain. Other treatments include physical therapy and wearing orthotic devices or shoe inserts. A doctor can also prescribe anti-inflammatory drugs and cortisone injections for pain. Sometimes surgery is needed to relieve the pressure and repair the toe joint.

Ingrown toenails occur when a piece of the nail breaks the skin—which can happen if you don't cut your nails properly. Ingrown toenails are very common in the large toes. A doctor can remove the part of the nail that is cutting into the skin. This allows the area to heal. Ingrown toenails can often be avoided by cutting the toenail straight across and level with the top of the toe.

Hammertoe is caused by a shortening of the tendons that control toe movements. The toe knuckle is usually enlarged, drawing the toe back. Over time, the joint enlarges and stiffens as it rubs against shoes. Your balance may be affected. Wearing shoes and stockings with plenty of toe room is a treatment for hammertoe. In very serious cases, surgery may be needed.

Spurs are calcium growths that develop on bones of your feet. They are caused by muscle strain in the feet. Standing for long periods of time, wearing badly fitting shoes, or being overweight can make spurs worse. Sometimes spurs are completely painless—at other times they can be very painful. Treatments for spurs include using foot supports, heel pads, and heel cups. Sometimes surgery is needed.

For More Information

For more information on foot care, contact:

American Podiatric Medical Association
9312 Old Georgetown Road
Bethesda, MD 20814
800-366-8227 (toll-free)
www.apma.org

American Orthopaedic Foot and Ankle Society
2517 Eastlake Avenue, East
Suite 200
Seattle, WA 98102
800-235-4855
www.aofas.org

For more information about health and aging, contact:

National Institute on Aging Information Center
P.O. Box 8057
Gaithersburg, MD 20898-8057
800-222-2225 (toll-free)
800-222-4225 (TTY/toll-free)

- To order publications (in English or Spanish) online, visit www.niapublications.org.
- The National Institute on Aging website is www.nia.nih.gov.

- Visit NIHSeniorHealth.gov (www.nihseniorhealth.gov), a senior-friendly website from the National Institute on Aging and the National Library of Medicine. This simple-to-use website features popular health topics for older adults. It has large type and a "talking" function that reads the text out loud.

May 2000

Good Nutrition: It's A Way of Life

"I have trouble chewing."

"Food just doesn't taste the same anymore."

"I don't have a car to go shopping."

"It's hard to cook for one person."

"I'm just not that hungry anymore."

Sound familiar? These are some of the common reasons older people stop eating right. And that's a problem because food provides energy and *nutrients* everyone needs to stay healthy. Nutrients include proteins, carbohydrates, fats, vitamins, minerals, and water. As you grow older, you may need less energy from what you eat. But, you still need just as many of the nutrients in food.

drinks with a lot of calories, but not many nutrients—for example, chips, cookies, sodas, and alcohol.

Calories are a way to measure the energy you get from food. If you eat more calories than your body needs, you could gain weight. Most packaged foods have the calorie counts listed on the labels.

What Should I Eat?

Choose many different healthy foods. Pick those that are lower in cholesterol and fat, especially saturated fat (mostly in foods that come from animals) and *trans fatty acids* (found in some processed foods, margarines, and shortenings). Avoid "empty calories" as much as you can. These are foods and

How Much Should I Eat?

The Dietary Guidelines from the U.S. Department of Agriculture (USDA) encourage people to eat a suggested amount from five major food groups every day. If you can't do that, at least try to eat something from each group each day. Lower fat choices are best. Make sure you include

GOOD NUTRITION: IT'S A WAY OF LIFE   **91**

vegetables, fruits, and whole-grain foods. Eating the smallest amount suggested will give you about 1,600 calories a day, the largest number has about 2,800 calories.

The Dietary Guidelines suggest:

Grains—5-10 ounces; some choices are:

- One roll, slice of bread, or small muffin,
- ½ cup of cooked rice or pasta, or
- About 1 cup (1 ounce) of ready-to-eat cereal.

Vegetables—2 to 3½ cups with a variety of colors and types of vegetables

Fruits—1½ to 2½ cups

Milk, yogurt, and cheese—3 cups of milk:

- 1 cup of yogurt equals 1 cup of milk,
- 1½ to 2 ounces of cheese equals 1 cup of milk, or
- 1 cup of cottage cheese equals ½ cup of milk.

Meat, poultry, fish, dry beans, eggs, and nuts—5 to 7 ounces of lean meat, poultry, or fish:

- ¼ cup of cooked beans or tofu, 1 egg, ½ ounce of nut or seeds, or 1 tablespoon of peanut butter—each can count as 1 ounce of meat.

How Many Calories Each Day for People Over Age 50?

A WOMAN:

- 1,600 calories, if her physical activity level is low
- 1,800 calories, if she is moderately active
- 2,000-2,200 calories if she has an active lifestyle

A MAN:

- 2,000 calories, if his physical activity level is low
- 2,200-2,400 calories, if he is moderately active
- 2,400-2,800 calories, if he has an active lifestyle

The more physically active you are, the more you might be able to eat without gaining weight.

Most people should have at least 30 minutes of moderate physical activity on most days of the week. Regular physical activity will help all areas of your life as you grow older.

Some other tips:

- Each day eat only small amounts of fats, oils, and sweets.
- When eating foods from the grains group, try to include at least 3 ounces from whole grains.
- Sometimes manufacturers put more than one serving in a package or bottle.

Another eating plan suggested by the Dietary Guidelines is called the DASH Eating Plan. DASH stands for Dietary Approaches to Stop Hypertension. See the resources at the end of this *Age Page* for more information on DASH.

Are You Less Interested in Food?

Does your favorite chicken dish taste different? Does Aunt Molly's pea soup suddenly seem to need salt? The flavor of the food is probably the same as always. With age your sense of taste and sense of smell may change. This affects how foods taste. They may seem to have lost flavor.

There are other reasons food may not taste the same. Some medicines can change your sense of taste or make you feel less hungry. Maybe you have slowed down a bit, so your body needs fewer calories. Maybe chewing is difficult because your dentures need to be adjusted or your teeth or gums need to be checked. You might want to pick softer foods to eat.

Do I Need to Drink Water?

Not just water. You need to drink plenty of liquids like water, juice, milk, and soup. You have to replace the fluids you lose every day. But check with your doctor if he or she has told you to limit how much you drink.

Don't wait until you feel thirsty to start drinking. With age you may lose some of your sense of thirst. In addition, medicine can sometimes cause you to lose fluids. If you are drinking enough, your urine will be pale yellow. If it is a bright or dark yellow, you need to drink more liquids.

Do you have a urinary control problem? If your answer is yes, don't stop drinking a lot of liquid. But, talk to your doctor for help with your urinary control problem.

What About Fiber?

Dietary fiber is found in foods that come from plants—fruits, vegetables, beans, nuts, seeds, brown rice, and whole grains. It is the part of plant foods that your body cannot digest. Eating more fiber might help you avoid intestinal problems like constipation, diverticulosis, and diverticulitis. It might also lower cholesterol and blood sugar and help you have regular bowel movements.

If you are not used to eating a lot of fiber, add more fiber to your diet slowly

GOOD NUTRITION: IT'S A WAY OF LIFE

to avoid stomach problems. The best source of this fiber is food, rather than dietary supplements. When adding fiber, remember:

- Eat cooked dry beans, peas, and lentils often.
- Leave skins on your fruit and vegetables if possible.
- Choose whole fruit over fruit juice.
- Eat whole-grain breads and cereals.
- Drink lots of fluids to help the fiber move through your intestines.

Should I Cut Back on Salt?

Salt (sodium chloride) is the most common way people get sodium. Sodium is naturally present in most foods, and salt is added to many canned and prepared foods. The body uses sodium to keep the blood, muscles, and nerves healthy. Too much is not good, however, and can make your blood pressure go up.

Most people eat a lot more sodium than they need. If you are over age 50, aim for 1,500 mg of sodium—about 2/3 of a teaspoon of table salt. That includes all the sodium you get in your food and drink, not just what you add when cooking or eating. If your doctor tells you to use less salt, cut back on salty snacks and processed foods. Try adding spices, herbs, and lemon juice to add flavor to your food. Also make sure your diet is rich in foods containing potassium. That will help counter the effects of salt on your blood pressure. Some foods that have a lot of potassium are leafy green vegetables, fruit from vines like tomatoes, bananas, and root vegetables like potatoes.

What About Fat?

Fat in your diet gives you energy and certain vitamins. But too much fat can be bad for your heart and blood vessels and can lead to heart disease. Fat is also high in calories.

To lower the fat in your diet:

- Choose lean cuts of meat, fish, or poultry (with the skin removed).
- Trim off any extra fat before cooking.
- Use low-fat dairy products and salad dressings.
- Use non-stick pots and pans, and cook without added fat.
- If you do use fat, use either an unsaturated vegetable oil or a nonfat cooking spray.
- Broil, roast, bake, stir-fry, steam, microwave, or boil foods. Avoid frying them.
- Season your foods with lemon juice, herbs, or spices, instead of butter.

What about Food Safety?

Because your sense of taste and smell may not work as well as you get older, you may not always be able to tell if foods have gone bad. You might want to date foods in your refrigerator to keep yourself from eating foods that are no longer fresh. If in doubt, throw it out.

Older people should be very careful with certain kinds of foods that need to be well cooked to prevent disease. For example, be sure to fully cook eggs, pork, fish, shellfish, poultry, and hot dogs. You might want to talk to your doctor or a registered dietitian, a specialist trained in nutrition, about foods you should avoid. These might include raw sprouts, some deli meats, and foods that are not *pasteurized* (heated enough to destroy disease-causing organisms), including some milk products.

Confused About What to Eat?

The USDA Dietary Guidelines suggest how much the "average" older person needs to eat. But, how does "average" match your needs? For example, maybe you have high cholesterol and need to keep a close eye on how much fat you eat. Or, possibly you have a food allergy or diabetes. Then you should check with your doctor or a dietitian. They can help you plan meals that will include the healthy foods you need without the foods you should not eat.

How Can I Make Shopping Easier?

Plan your meals in advance. Check your supply of staples like flour, sugar, rice, and cereal. Make a list of what you need. Keep some canned or frozen foods on hand. These are handy when you do not feel like cooking or cannot go out. Powdered nonfat dry milk, canned evaporated milk, and ultra-pasteurized milk in a carton can be stored easily.

Think about how much of a product you will use. A large size may be cheaper per unit, but it is not a bargain if you end up throwing much of it away. Share large packages with a friend. Frozen vegetables sold in bags save money because you can use small amounts while keeping the rest frozen. If a package of meat or fresh produce is too large, ask a store employee to repackage it in a smaller size.

Learn to read food package labels. There, you will find a list of ingredients. The first one listed is present in the food in the largest amount. The ones that follow are present in smaller and smaller amounts. Look at "Nutrition Facts" for the calories, protein, carbohydrate, fat, sodium, fiber, vitamin, and mineral amounts per serving. The label also suggests a serving size for comparing foods. There may be an expiration or "use by" date on the label or container. At

GOOD NUTRITION: IT'S A WAY OF LIFE

first, reading labels will add some time to your shopping trip. Soon you will learn which products are best for you.

Won't All This Food Cost A Lot?

Here are some ways to keep your food costs down:

- Plain (generic) labels, if available, or store brands are usually cheaper than name brands.
- Plan your menu around items on sale.
- Prepare more of the foods you enjoy, and quickly refrigerate the leftovers to eat in a day or two.
- Divide leftovers into individual servings. Write the contents and date on each package, and freeze to use within a few months.
- Share meal preparation and costs with a friend.
- Plan a "pot-luck" dinner where everyone brings a prepared dish.

Food stamps from the Federal Government help people with low incomes buy groceries. If you think you are eligible, check with a local food stamps office or Area Agency on Aging. Also ask your local Area Agency on Aging or tribal organization about the nearest senior center or nutrition site. You may be able to enjoy free or low-cost meals for older people at a community center, church, or school. These meals offer good food and a chance to be with other people. Home delivered meals are available for people who are homebound.

For More Information

To learn more about nutrition, meal programs, or help with shopping, contact:

Administration on Aging
330 Independence Avenue, SW
Washington, DC 20201
202-619-7501
www.aoa.gov

- Eldercare Locator:
  800-677-1116 (toll-free)
  www.eldercare.gov

USDA Food and Nutrition Information Center (FNIC)
10301 Baltimore Avenue
Room 304
Beltsville, MD 20705-2351
301-504-5719
www.nal.usda.gov/fnic

To learn about DASH, go to:

National Heart, Lung, and Blood Institute
P.O. Box 30105
Bethesda, MD 20824-0105
301-592-8573
240-629-3255 (TTY)
www.nhlbi.nih.gov

The federal government has three websites with information on nutrition:

www.nutrition.gov
www.healthierus.gov
www.mypyramid.gov

For more information about health, exercise, and aging, contact:

National Institute on Aging Information Center
P.O. Box 8057
Gaithersburg, MD 20898-8057
800-222-2225 (toll-free)
800-222-4225 (TTY/toll-free)

- To order publications (in English or Spanish) online, visit *www.niapublications.org*.
- The National Institute on Aging website is *www.nia.nih.gov*.
- Visit NIHSeniorHealth.gov (*www.nihseniorhealth.gov*), a senior-friendly website from the National Institute on Aging and the National Library of Medicine. This simple-to-use website features popular health topics for older adults. It has large type and a "talking" function that reads the text out loud.

April 2005

Life Extension: Science Fact or Science Fiction?

> Bill just died of a heart attack at age 67. His brother, Jim, 12 years older, still enjoys playing golf once a week. Why is Jim living so much longer? Does he take after their mother's family who all lived into their eighties? Or, does he just have a healthier lifestyle?

What makes people grow old? How can we live longer? Why do members of some families seem to live longer than others? Can people live to 150 years old? Would you want to? These questions have fascinated people for centuries. Now scientists who study aging, called gerontologists, are trying to answer them.

Genes now being studied may one day answer some of these questions. Genes might be considered little packets of information found in each cell in our bodies. These packets contain instructions that tell our bodies how to grow and work. For example, they control whether we get our grandmother's blue eyes or our father's crooked little finger. For some people genes may affect how long they live.

Areas of Research

Several "longevity genes" have been found in some living organisms. Scientists studying certain worms and fruit flies have found several genes that seem to control how long these creatures live. By making a change in just one of these genes, they have almost doubled the average lifespan of both fruit flies and one type of worm. Others looking at longevity genes have shown that the gene already shown to control how fast yeast cells age may do the same thing in mice. This gene is also present in humans. As interesting as this work is, it is unlikely that changing genes will be tried in humans in the near future as a way to help them live longer.

Genes alone, however, are only a part of the reason that some people live a long time. How people live, their lifestyle, may be more important. For example, does someone smoke? Do they exercise? Are they under a lot of stress? What do they eat? Some scientists think what people eat and how much they eat can lead to a longer life. Caloric restriction is one area of research on aging. A calorie-restricted diet has 30 to 40% fewer calories than a normal diet, but it has all the needed nutrients. This diet seems to extend the life of almost every animal type in which it is studied. It has worked in protozoa (very small, one-celled organisms), fruit flies, mice, and rats. Recent studies in primates, such as monkeys, are not complete. They do, however, show a slowing in some measures of the aging process in primates on this diet. Primates are our closest animal relatives. This diet has not been tested in humans. We do not know whether it will have the same life-extending effect in people. Conducting such a study in people is not practical because people would have trouble following such a diet.

How does caloric restriction work? We do not know. Some scientists think that eating fewer calories lowers body temperature and changes metabolism, the breakdown of substances so that the body can easily use them. This, in turn, lessens damage to cells and slows certain other cell-damaging activities. In fact, caloric restriction seems to slow the whole process of growing older. Animals that have been on restricted diets since their youth reach adulthood later than others not on these diets. Not only do these animals seem to live longer, they also have less illness. Although we don't know how this works in people, scientists do know the flipside—that people who are overweight are more likely to develop certain age-related diseases such as heart and blood vessel disease, high blood pressure, arthritis, cancer, and diabetes.

Is there is a link between the so-called longevity genes and our body's use of food? The single gene in fruit flies that was changed to lengthen their lifespan is related to the way that the fruit fly stores and uses energy, usually gotten from food. Other scientists studying genes in yeast cells recently found a chemical that seems to work with a longevity gene to increase the yeast cell's lifespan. This chemical is also part of the yeast cell's processing of energy.

Experts in aging do not expect ever to recommend such caloric restriction for people. But these studies will help them understand aging. They may also teach us how to prevent or delay diseases that seem to come with growing older. Understanding how caloric restriction works might also help scientists develop chemicals that could imitate its effects on the aging process.

Looking for a Youth Pill

Many people hope research will point the way to a fountain of youth. Or, perhaps a modern-day magic potion to slow the aging process and keep people younger longer. But, before scientists can hope to do this, they must first learn how and why we age.

Investigators have begun to find certain chemicals such as hormones in our bodies that change as we age. Levels of some substances fall as we grow older. It's easy to see how some people might think that if we replace these chemicals, we could slow, stop, or even reverse aging. Some stores, catalogs, and Internet websites now sell products that are similar to these chemicals. However, the advertising claims that these products can extend life or make you feel younger are not proven.

Antioxidants

Antioxidants are natural substances in foods. They may help protect you from disease by preventing the harmful effects of *oxygen free radicals* on your body. Oxygen free radicals are formed as cells in your body combine with oxygen to make energy. Free radicals also come from smoking or being exposed to things in the environment like radiation or sunlight. As we age, this damage may build up. According to one theory of aging, in time this build-up harms cells, tissues, and organs.

Your body's own antioxidant defense system stops most free-radical damage, but not all. Antioxidants may prevent cataracts and heart disease, protect against damage from smoking, or boost immunity to illness.

Some antioxidants, such as the enzyme SOD (superoxide dismutase), are only useful when produced in the body. SOD pills have no effect on the body. They are broken up into different substances during digestion. Other antioxidants that come from food include:

- Beta-carotene, present in deep-colored fruits and vegetables,
- Selenium, found in seafood, liver, meat, and grains,
- Vitamin C, from citrus fruits, peppers, tomatoes, and berries, and
- Vitamin E, present in wheat germ, nuts, sesame seeds, and canola, olive, and peanut oils.

How much of these antioxidants should you use, if at all? The National Academy of Sciences is a nongovernmental group of experts involved in scientific research. They recommend what vitamins and minerals you need in your diet and how much of each. They say that there is no proof that large doses of antioxidants will prevent chronic diseases such as heart disease, diabetes, or cataracts. They did set guidelines for the safe use of some of them:

- Selenium—at least 55 micrograms (mcg) per day but not more than 400 mcg per day.
- Vitamin C—at least 75 milligrams (mg) per day for women and 90 mg for men, although smokers need more. No one should have more than 2,000 mg per day.
- Vitamin E—at least 15 mg per day from food and not more than 1,000 mg per day.

DHEA

DHEA is short for dehydroepiandrosterone. This is a hormone that has modified some age-related changes in animals. When given to mice, it boosted some components of the immune system and helped prevent some kinds of cancer. Several studies in older people have shown that DHEA helps build muscle, but other studies have not agreed. Some people hope DHEA will improve energy and immunity, increase muscles, and decrease body fat, but there is not enough research to support these claims or even to show that taking DHEA is safe.

DHEA travels through the bloodstream in a special form called DHEA sulfate. It turns into DHEA when it enters a cell. Levels of DHEA sulfate are high in younger people but tend to go down with age. The body changes DHEA into two other strong hormones: estrogen and testosterone. Taking DHEA supplements can cause some people's bodies to make large amounts of these two hormones. This could be dangerous. High levels of naturally made testosterone in men and estrogen in women may play a role in prostate cancer in men and breast cancer in women. Experts do not know if supplements of DHEA will increase your chance of developing these cancers.

Growth Hormone

Similar claims of more energy and muscle strength and less body fat are also made for human growth hormone (hGH) supplements. This hormone is made naturally by the pituitary gland. Children need hGH to grow normally. It also helps keep our tissues and organs healthy. Our bodies make less hGH as we age.

The only approved use for hGH is a shot given to children whose bodies do not make enough growth hormone. Only doctors may prescribe and give hGH shots. Despite this, some people spend thousands of dollars a year on these shots because they hope to slow down their bodies' aging. Others, who cannot afford the injections, buy over-the-counter "hGH releasers." Claims that these releasers will make the body "release" more hGH are unproven.

What scientists do know is that in recent studies injections of growth hormone for a short time seemed to boost the size and strength of muscles and to lessen body fat in a small group of older men and women. Adding testosterone increased these benefits in men. Using estrogen did not bring about further muscle and body fat changes in women. Longer studies with larger numbers of older people are needed to find out if hGH can prevent weakness and frailty in older people without causing dangerous side effects.

What harm might using hGH for longer periods of time do? Some experts believe that such hGH treatment can lead to diabetes, the collection of fluid in body tissues, and carpal tunnel syndrome. Some of these side effects may be very serious in older adults. If the body makes too much growth hormone during adulthood, certain tissues, such as bones, may grow more than they are supposed to. This condition is called *acromegaly*. Scientists

LIFE EXTENSION: SCIENCE FACT OR SCIENCE FICTION?

do not know if too much supplementation with growth hormone in adults could cause a similar problem.

Dietary Supplements

Dietary supplements are now sold in almost every shopping mall, grocery store, drug store, and convenience store, as well as on the Web. Each year people spend billions of dollars on these vitamins, minerals, herbs, and hormones. They are hoping for more energy, stronger muscles, better memory, protection from disease, and maybe even a longer life. The Food and Drug Administration (FDA) does not oversee most of these products. So you can't be sure that a supplement's health claims are true or that they are safe to take for a long period of time. You cannot even be sure that the preparations are pure or consistent from bottle-to-bottle, or manufacturer-to-manufacturer.

Some of the more common dietary supplements include ginkgo biloba, ginseng, saw palmetto, Echinacea, and St. John's wort. Although there may be a lot of word-of-mouth talk about these supplements, we don't know the truth. Several of these herbal remedies offer hope for treating health problems in the elderly. However, more research in older people needs to be done before experts can recommend any products. There are still a lot of questions about consumer safety.

The Bottom Line

It may be that the basic question is "how can I stay healthy and independent as I grow older?" Right now there are no treatments, drugs, or pills known to slow aging or extend human life. Check with your doctor before buying pills or anything else that promises to do such things or to make a big change in the way you look or feel. These purchases might be unsafe or a waste of money. They might even interfere with other treatments you are already receiving.

Ten Tips for Healthy Aging

No substance can extend life, but the chances of staying healthy and living longer can be improved if you:

- Eat a balanced diet, including five helpings of fruits and vegetables a day.
- Exercise regularly (check with a doctor before starting an exercise program if you have any chronic illnesses).
- Get regular health checkups.
- Stop smoking (it's never too late to quit).
- Practice safety habits at home to prevent falls and fractures. Always wear your seatbelt in a car.
- Stay in contact with family and friends. Stay active through work, play, and community.
- Avoid overexposure to the sun and the cold.
- Use moderation if you drink alcohol. When you drink, let someone else drive.

- Keep personal and financial records in order to simplify budgeting and investing. Plan long-term housing and money needs.

- Keep a positive attitude toward life. Do things that make you happy.

For More Information

The National Institute on Aging offers a publication, *Pills, Patches, and Shots: Can Hormones Prevent Aging?*, which discusses the question of replacing hormones that decline naturally with age. For that or other information about health and aging, contact:

National Institute on Aging Information Center
P.O. Box 8057
Gaithersburg, MD 20898-8057
800-222-2225 (toll-free)
800-222-4225 (TTY/toll-free)

- To order publications (in English or Spanish) online, visit *www.niapublications.org*.

- The National Institute on Aging website is *www.nia.nih.gov*.

- Visit NIHSeniorHealth.gov (*www.nihseniorhealth.gov*), a senior-friendly website from the National Institute on Aging and the National Library of Medicine. This simple-to-use website features popular health topics for older adults. It has large type and a "talking" function that reads the text out loud.

July 2001

Sexuality in Later Life

People seem to want and need to be close to others. We want to share our thoughts and feelings with others and to touch and be touched. Just being physically near is important, but many of us also want to continue an active, satisfying sex life as we grow older. However, over time most people may find that it takes them longer to become sexually aroused. This is part of the normal aging process.

What Are Normal Changes?

Normal aging brings physical changes in both men and women. These changes sometimes affect one's ability to have and enjoy sex with another person.

Some women enjoy sex more as they grow older. After menopause or a hysterectomy, they may no longer fear an unwanted pregnancy. They may feel freer to enjoy sex. Some women do not think things like gray hair and wrinkles make them less attractive to their sexual partner. But if a woman believes that looking young or being able to give birth makes her more feminine, she may begin to worry about how desirable she is no matter what her age is. That might make sex less enjoyable for her.

A woman may notice changes in her vagina. As she ages, her vagina shortens and narrows. The walls become thinner and also a little stiffer. These changes do not mean she can't enjoy having sex. However, most women will also have less vaginal lubrication. This could affect sexual pleasure.

As men get older, impotence becomes more common. Impotence is the loss of ability to have and keep an erection hard enough for sexual intercourse. By age 65, about 15 to 25% of men have this problem at least one out of every four times they are having sex. This may happen in men with heart disease, high blood pressure, or diabetes—either because of the disease or the medicines used to treat it.

A man may find it takes longer to get an erection. His erection may not be as firm or as large as it used to be. The amount of ejaculate may be smaller. The loss of erection after orgasm may happen more quickly, or it may take longer before an erection is again possible. Some men may find they need more foreplay.

What Causes Sexual Problems?

Illness, disability, or the drugs you take to treat a health problem can affect your ability to have and enjoy sex. But, even the most serious health problems usually don't have to stop you from having a satisfying sex life.

Arthritis. Joint pain due to arthritis can make sexual contact uncomfortable. Joint replacement surgery and drugs may relieve this pain. Exercise, rest, warm baths, and changing the position or timing of sexual activity can be helpful.

Chronic pain. In addition to arthritis, pain that continues for more than a month or comes back on and off over time can be caused by other bone and muscle conditions, shingles, poor blood circulation, or blood vessel problems. This discomfort can, in turn, lead to sleep problems, depression, isolation, and difficulty moving around. These can interfere with intimacy between older people. Chronic pain does not have to be part of growing older and can often be treated.

Diabetes. Many men with diabetes do not have sexual problems, but this is one of the few illnesses that can cause impotence. In most cases medical treatment can help.

Heart disease. Narrowing and hardening of the arteries known as atherosclerosis can change blood vessels so that blood does not flow freely. This can lead to trouble with erections in men, as can high blood pressure (hypertension).

Some people who have had a heart attack are afraid that having sex will cause another attack. The chance of this is very low. Most people can start having sex again 3 to 6 weeks after their condition becomes stable following an attack, if their doctor agrees. Always follow your doctor's advice.

Incontinence. Loss of bladder control or leaking of urine is more common as we grow older, especially in women. Stress incontinence happens during exercise, coughing, sneezing, or lifting, for example. Because of the extra pressure on your abdomen during sex, incontinence might cause some people to avoid sex. The good news is that this can usually be treated.

Stroke. The ability to have sex is rarely damaged by a stroke, but problems with erections are possible. It is unlikely that having sex will cause another stroke. Someone with weakness or paralysis caused by a stroke might try using different positions or medical devices to help them continue having sex.

What About Surgery and Drugs?

Surgery. Many of us worry about having any kind of surgery—it is especially troubling when the genital area is involved. Happily, most people do return to the kind of sex life they enjoyed before having surgery.

Hysterectomy is surgery to remove the uterus. It does not interfere with sexual functioning. If a hysterectomy seems to take away from a woman's ability to enjoy sex, a counselor may be helpful. Men who feel their partners are "less feminine" after a hysterectomy may also be helped by counseling.

Mastectomy is surgery to remove all or part of a woman's breast. Your body is as capable of sexual response as ever, but you may lose your sexual desire or sense of being desired. Sometimes it is useful to talk with other women who have had this surgery. Programs like the American Cancer Society's (ACS) "Reach to Recovery" can be helpful for both women and men. Rebuilding of the breast (reconstruction) is also a possibility to discuss with your surgeon.

About 1,500 American men develop breast cancer each year. In them the disease can make their bodies make extra "female" hormones. These can greatly lower their sex drive.

Prostatectomy is surgery that removes all or part of a man's prostate. Sometimes this procedure is done because of an enlarged prostate. It may cause urinary incontinence or impotence. If removal of the prostate gland (radical prostatectomy) is needed, doctors can often save the nerves going to the penis. An erection may still be possible. Talk to your doctor before surgery to make sure you will be able to lead a fully satisfying sex life.

Medications. Some drugs can cause sexual problems. These include some blood pressure medicines, antihistamines, antidepressants, tranquilizers, appetite suppressants, diabetes drugs, and some ulcer drugs like ranitidine. Some can lead to impotence or make it hard for men to ejaculate. Some drugs can reduce a woman's sexual desire. Check with your doctor. She or he can often prescribe a different drug without this side effect.

Alcohol. Too much alcohol can cause erection problems in men and delay orgasm in women.

Am I Too Old to Worry About Safe Sex?

Having safe sex is important for people at any age. As a woman gets closer to menopause, her periods may be irregular. But, she can still get pregnant. In fact, pregnancy is still possible until your doctor says you are past menopause—you have not had a menstrual period for 12 months.

Age does not protect you from sexually transmitted diseases. Young people are most at risk for diseases such as syphilis, gonorrhea, chlamydial infection, genital herpes, hepatitis B, genital warts, and trichomoniasis. But these diseases can and do happen in sexually active older people.

Almost anyone who is sexually active is also at risk for being infected with HIV, the virus that causes AIDS. The number of older people with HIV/AIDS is growing. One out of every 10 people diagnosed with AIDS in the United States is over age 50. You are at risk if you have more than one sexual partner or are recently divorced or widowed and have started dating and having unprotected sex again. Always use a latex condom during sex, and talk to your doctor about ways to protect yourself from all sexually transmitted diseases. You are never too old to be at risk.

Can Emotions Play a Part?

Sexuality is often a delicate balance of emotional and physical issues. How you feel may affect what you are able to do. For example, men may fear that impotence will become a more common problem as they age. But, if you are too concerned with that possibility, you can cause enough stress to trigger impotence. A woman who is worried about how her looks are changing as she ages may think her partner will no longer find her attractive.

This focus on youthful physical beauty may get in the way of her enjoyment of sex.

Older couples face the same daily stresses that affect people of any age. But they may also have the added concerns of age, illness, and retirement and other lifestyle changes. These worries can cause sexual difficulties. Talk openly with your doctor, or see a counselor. These health professionals can often help.

Don't blame yourself for any sexual difficulties you and your partner are having. You might want to talk with a therapist about them. If your male partner is troubled by impotence or your female partner seems less interested in sex, don't assume they don't find you attractive anymore. There can be many physical causes for their problems.

What Can I Do?

There are several things you can do on your own to keep an active sexual life. Remember that sex does not have to include intercourse. Make your partner a high priority. Pay attention to his or her needs and wants. Take time to understand the changes you both are facing. Try different positions and new times, like having sex in the morning when you both may have more energy. Don't hurry—you or your partner may need to spend more time touching to become fully aroused. Masturbation is a sexual activity that some older people, especially unmarried, widowed, or divorced people and those whose partners are ill or away, may find satisfying.

Some older people, especially women, may have trouble finding a partner with whom they can share any type of intimacy. Women live longer than men, so there are more of them. In 2000, women over age 65 outnumbered older men by 100 to 70. Doing activities that other seniors enjoy or going places where older people gather are ways to meet new people. Some ideas include mall walking, senior centers, adult education classes at a community college, or day trips sponsored by your city or county recreation department.

If you do seem to have a problem that affects your sex life, talk to your doctor. He or she can suggest a treatment depending on the type of problem and its cause. For example, the most common sexual difficulty of older women is dyspareunia, painful intercourse caused by poor vaginal lubrication. Your doctor or a pharmacist can suggest over-the-counter, water-based vaginal lubricants to use. Or, your doctor might suggest estrogen supplements or an estrogen vaginal insert.

If impotence is the problem, it can often be managed and perhaps even reversed. There is a pill that can help. It is called sildenafil and should not be taken by men taking medicines containing nitrates, such as nitroglycerin. This pill does have possible side effects. Other available treatments include vacuum devices, self-injection of a drug (either papaverine or prostaglandin E1), or penile implants.

There is a lot you can do to continue an active sex life. Follow a healthy lifestyle—exercise, eat good food, drink plenty of fluids like water or juices, don't smoke, and avoid alcohol. Try to reduce the stress in your life. See your doctor regularly. And keep a positive outlook on life.

For More Information

The following organizations and government agencies have information that may be of help:

American Cancer Society
1599 Clifton Road, NE
Atlanta, GA 30329
800-227-2345 (toll-free)
www.cancer.org

American Urological Association Foundation, Inc.
1000 Corporate Boulevard
Linthicum, MD 21090
866-746-4282 (toll-free)
410-689-6700
www.urologyhealth.org

National Institute of Diabetes and Digestive and Kidney Diseases
National Kidney and Urologic Diseases Information Clearinghouse
3 Information Way
Bethesda, MD 20892-3580
800-891-5390 (toll-free)
301-654-4415
www.niddk.nih.gov

For more information about health and aging, contact:

National Institute on Aging Information Center
P.O. Box 8057
Gaithersburg, MD 20898-8057
800-222-2225 (toll-free)
800-222-4225 (TTY/toll-free)

- To order publications (in English or Spanish) online, visit www.niapublications.org.

- The National Institute on Aging website is www.nia.nih.gov.

- Visit NIHSeniorHealth.gov (www.nihseniorhealth.gov), a senior-friendly website from the National Institute on Aging and the National Library of Medicine. This simple-to-use website features popular health topics for older adults. It has large type and a "talking" function that reads the text out loud.

August 2002

Shots for Safety

Shots—or immunizations—are not just for children! Adults also need to be vaccinated from time to time to protect themselves against serious infectious diseases. In fact, some shots are more important for adults than for children. Every year, thousands of older people die needlessly. The Federal Government's Centers for Disease Control and Prevention (CDC) strongly encourage older adults to be immunized against flu, pneumococcal disease, tetanus and diphtheria, and chickenpox, as well as measles, mumps, and rubella.

Flu

Flu—the short name for influenza—is a highly contagious infection that causes fever, chills, dry cough, sore throat, runny or stuffy nose, as well as headache, muscle aches, and often extreme fatigue. Flu usually is a mild disease in healthy children, young adults, and middle-aged people. However, it can be life threatening in older adults.

Flu viruses change all the time. For this reason, you need to get a flu shot every year. To give your body time to build the proper defense, it's important to get a flu shot between September and mid-November, before the flu season usually starts.

Although side effects from the flu shot are slight for most people, some soreness, redness, or swelling may occur on the arm where the shot was given. About 5 to 10% of people have mild side effects such as headache or low-grade fever, which last for about a day after vaccination.

The flu shot is the primary method of preventing and controlling the flu. However, four drugs have been approved to treat people who get the flu: amantadine (Symmetrel), rimantadine (Flumadine), zanamivir (Relenza), and oseltamivir (Tamiflu). When taken within 48 hours after the onset of illness, these drugs reduce the duration of fever and other symptoms. These drugs are available only by prescription.

Pneumococcal Disease

Pneumococcal disease is a serious infection. Many people are familiar with pneumococcal pneumonia, which affects the lungs. But the bacteria that cause this form of pneumonia also can attack other parts of the body. When the same bacteria invade the lining of the brain, they cause meningitis. When they enter the bloodstream, they cause bacteremia. They also can cause middle ear and sinus infections.

The CDC recommends that people 65 and older get the pneumococcal vaccine. The shot is safe and can be given at the same time as the flu shot. Most people only need a single dose. However, the CDC advises people 65 and older to have a second dose of the pneumococcal vaccine if they received the shot more than five years previously and were younger than 65 when they were vaccinated the first time. No one should receive more than two total doses of the pneumococcal vaccine available now.

About half of the people who get the shot have minor side effects—temporary swelling, redness, and soreness at the place on the arm where the shot was given. A few people (less than 1 percent) have fever, muscle pain, or more serious swelling and pain on the arm.

Pneumococcal disease is treated with antibiotics. However, in recent years the bacteria that cause pneumococcal disease have become more and more resistant to penicillin. This is one reason why prevention and the development of newer, more effective vaccines are so important.

Tetanus and Diphtheria

Tetanus (sometimes called lockjaw) is caused by the toxin (poison) of a bacterium. The bacteria can enter the body through a tiny pinprick or scratch but prefer deep puncture wounds or cuts like those made by nails or knives. Tetanus bacteria commonly are found in soil, dust, and manure. Tetanus is not spread from person to person. Common first signs of tetanus are headache and muscle stiffness in the jaw, followed by stiffness of the neck, difficulty swallowing, muscle spasms, sweating, and fever.

Diphtheria usually affects the tonsils, throat, nose, or skin. Like tetanus, it is caused by the toxin, or poison, of a bacterium, but it can spread from an infected person to the nose or throat of others. It can lead to breathing problems, heart failure, paralysis, and sometimes death. Diphtheria may be mistaken for a severe sore throat. Other symptoms include a low-grade fever and enlarged lymph nodes in the neck. A second form of diphtheria causes sores on the skin that may be painful, red, and swollen.

Vaccination is the best way to protect yourself against tetanus and diphtheria. Most people receive their first vaccine as children in the form of a combined diphtheria-tetanus-pertussis vaccine or DTP. For adults, a combination shot, called a Td booster, protects against both tetanus and diphtheria. You need a Td shot every 10 years throughout life to protect yourself against these rare, but dangerous, illnesses. During everyday activities (such as gardening), the tetanus bacteria can enter a break in the skin and cause infection. It's particularly important to have a booster shot if you have a severe cut or puncture wound and haven't had a booster in the past 5 to 10 years.

The Td vaccine is safe and effective. Most people have no problems with it. When side effects do occur, they usually are minor and include soreness, redness, or swelling on the arm where the shot was given.

Chickenpox

Chickenpox—also known as varicella—is a very contagious disease that is caused by a virus. It is spread easily through the air by infected people when they sneeze or cough. The disease also spreads through contact with an infected person's chickenpox sores. People who have never had chickenpox can get infected just by being in the room with someone who has the disease.

While chickenpox is a mild disease for children, adults usually get much sicker. Early symptoms include aching, tiredness, fever, and sore throat. Then, an itchy, blister-like rash appears.

People who have had chickenpox are protected from getting it again. A vaccine is available to protect people who have not had chickenpox. Two doses of the vaccine are recommended for people 13 years of age and older. Most people who get chickenpox vaccine don't have problems with it. The most common side effects are mild and include pain and swelling on the arm where the shot was given. Fever or a mild rash may develop.

Some people who have had chickenpox may develop shingles later in life. Shingles is caused by a reactivation of the same virus that produces chickenpox.

The National Institute of Allergy and Infectious Diseases has tested a shingles vaccine. The vaccine is similar to the one used to immunize against chickenpox. Scientists hope that this adult vaccine to prevent shingles will be available in the future.

Measles, Mumps, and Rubella

Measles, mumps, and rubella were once very common diseases in the United States, but they have become rare because of the use of vaccines to prevent them. As with many other diseases, measles, mumps, and rubella generally are more severe in adults than in children. Most adults are immune to all three infections because they had them (or a vaccine) as children.

SHOTS FOR SAFETY **111**

Everyone born in or after 1957 should have received at least one dose of the measles-mumps-rubella (MMR) vaccine sometime after their first birthday. Some adults—such as health care workers and people who travel out of the United States—may need a second dose. People born before 1957 may be vaccinated if they believe they've never had one of these diseases. There's no harm in receiving the vaccine if you already are immune to the infection.

Travel

If you are planning to travel abroad, check with your doctor or local health department about the shots that you need. Sometimes a series of shots is needed, so it's best to get them well in advance of your trip. For information about specific vaccines required by different countries, general health measures for travelers, and reported outbreaks, call the CDC information line for international travelers at 877-394-8747. The website address is *www.cdc.gov/travel*.

Keeping a Shot Record

It's helpful to keep a personal immunization record with the types and dates of shots you've received, as well as any side effects or problems that you had. The medical record in your doctor's office also should be kept up to date.

Widespread use of vaccines can reduce the risk of developing a number of contagious diseases that seriously affect older people. You can protect yourself against these illnesses by including vaccinations as part of your regular health care.

For More Information

Information about adult immunizations also is available from the following groups:

National Institute of Allergy and Infectious Diseases
301-496-5717
www.niaid.nih.gov

Centers for Disease Control and Prevention
National Immunization Information Hotline
800-232-4636 (toll-free)
www.cdc.gov

American Lung Association
800-586-4872 (toll-free)
www.lungusa.org

National Coalition for Adult Immunization
4733 Bethesda Avenue
Suite 750
Bethesda, MD 20814
www.nfid.org/ncai

For more information about health and aging, contact:

National Institute on Aging Information Center
P.O. Box 8057
Gaithersburg, MD 20898-8057
800-222-2225 (toll-free)
800-222-4225 (TTY/toll-free)

- To order publications (in English or Spanish) online, visit *www.niapublications.org*.
- The National Institute on Aging website is *www.nia.nih.gov*.
- Visit NIHSeniorHealth.gov (*www.nihseniorhealth.gov*), a senior-friendly website from the National Institute on Aging and the National Library of Medicine. This simple-to-use website features popular health topics for older adults. It has large type and a "talking" function that reads the text out loud.

April 2000

SHOTS FOR SAFETY 113

Skin Care and Aging

> "Defy aging."
>
> "Tone and firm sagging skin."
>
> "Restore your skin's own wrinkle control."

Americans spend billions of dollars each year on skin care products that promise to erase wrinkles, lighten age spots, and eliminate itching, flaking, or redness. But the simplest and cheapest way to keep your skin healthy and young looking is to stay out of the sun.

Sunlight is a major cause of the skin changes we think of as aging—changes such as wrinkles, dryness, and age spots. Your skin does change with age. For example, you sweat less, leading to increased dryness. As your skin ages, it becomes thinner and loses fat, so it looks less plump and smooth. Underlying structures—veins and bones in particular—become more prominent. Your skin can take longer to heal when injured.

You can delay these changes by staying out of the sun. Although nothing can completely undo sun damage, the skin sometimes can repair itself. So, it's never too late to protect yourself from the harmful effects of the sun.

Wrinkles

Over time, the sun's ultraviolet (UV) light damages the fibers in the skin called elastin. The breakdown of these fibers causes the skin to lose its ability to snap back after stretching. As a result, wrinkles form. Gravity also is at work, pulling at the skin and causing it to sag, most noticeably on the face, neck, and upper arms.

Cigarette smoking also contributes to wrinkles. People who smoke tend to have more wrinkles than nonsmokers of the same age, complexion, and history of sun exposure. The reason for this difference is not clear. It may be because smoking also plays a role in damaging elastin. Facial wrinkling increases with the amount of cigarettes and number of years a person has smoked.

Many products currently on the market claim to "revitalize aging skin." According to the American Academy of Dermatology, over-the-counter "wrinkle" creams and

114 BOUND FOR YOUR GOOD HEALTH: A COLLECTION OF AGE PAGES

lotions may soothe dry skin, but they do little or nothing to reverse wrinkles. At this time, the only products that have been studied for safety and effectiveness and approved by the Food and Drug Administration (FDA) to treat signs of sun-damaged or aging skin are tretinoin cream and carbon dioxide (CO_2) and erbium (Er:YAG) lasers.

Tretinoin cream (Renova), a vitamin A derivative available by prescription only, is approved for reducing the appearance of fine wrinkles, mottled darkened spots, and roughness in people whose skin doesn't improve with regular skin care and use of sun protection. However, it doesn't eliminate wrinkles, repair sun-damaged skin, or restore skin to its healthier, younger structure. It hasn't been studied in people 50 and older or in people with moderately or darkly pigmented skin.

The CO_2 and Er:YAG lasers are approved to treat wrinkles. The doctor uses the laser to remove skin one layer at a time. Laser therapy is performed under anesthesia in an outpatient surgical setting.

The FDA currently is studying the safety of alpha hydroxy acids (AHAs), which are widely promoted to reduce wrinkles, spots, and other signs of aging, sun-damaged skin. Some studies suggest that they may work, but there is concern about adverse reactions and long-term effects of their use. Because people who use AHA products have greater sensitivity to the sun, the FDA advises consumers to protect themselves from sun exposure by using sunscreen, wearing a hat, or avoiding mid-day sun. If you are interested in treatment for wrinkles, you should discuss treatment options with a dermatologist.

Dry Skin and Itching

Many older people suffer from dry skin, particularly on their lower legs, elbows, and forearms. The skin feels rough and scaly and often is accompanied by a distressing, intense itchiness. Low humidity—caused by overheating during the winter and air conditioning during the summer—contributes to dryness and itching. The loss of sweat and oil glands as you age also may worsen dry skin. Anything that further dries your skin—such as overuse of soaps, antiperspirants, perfumes, or hot baths—will make the problem worse. Dehydration, sun exposure, smoking, and stress also may cause dry skin.

Dry skin itches because it is irritated easily. If your skin is very dry and itchy, see a doctor. Dry skin and itching can affect your sleep, cause irritability, or be a symptom of a disease. For example, diabetes and kidney disease can cause itching. Some medicines make the itchiness worse.

The most common treatment for dry skin is the use of moisturizers to reduce water loss and soothe the skin. Moisturizers come in several forms—ointments, creams, and lotions. *Ointments* are mixtures of water in oil, usually either lanolin or petrolatum. *Creams* are preparations of oil in water, which is the main ingredient. Creams must be applied more often than ointments to be most effective. *Lotions* contain powder crystals dissolved in water, again the main ingredient. Because of their high water content, they feel cool on the skin and don't leave the skin feeling greasy. Although they are easy to apply and may be more pleasing than ointments and creams, lotions don't have the same protective qualities. You may need to apply them frequently to relieve the signs and symptoms of dryness. Moisturizers should be used indefinitely to prevent recurrence of dry skin.

A humidifier can add moisture to the air. Bathing less often and using milder soaps also can help relieve dry skin. Warm water is less irritating to dry skin than hot water.

Skin Cancer

Skin cancer is the most common type of cancer in the United States. According to current estimates, 40 to 50% of Americans who live to age 65 will have skin cancer at least once. Although anyone can get skin cancer, the risk is greatest for people who have fair skin that freckles easily.

UV radiation from the sun is the main cause of skin cancer. In addition, artificial sources of UV radiation—such as sunlamps and tanning booths—can cause skin cancer. People who live in areas of the United States that get high levels of UV radiation from the sun are more likely to get skin cancer. For example, skin cancer is more common in Texas and Florida than in Minnesota, where the sun is not as strong.

There are three common types of skin cancers. *Basal cell carcinomas* are the most common, accounting for more than 90 percent of all skin cancers in the United States. They are slow-growing cancers that seldom spread to other parts of the body. *Squamous cell carcinomas* also rarely spread, but they do so more often than basal cell carcinomas. The most dangerous of all cancers that occur in the skin is *melanoma*. Melanoma can spread to other organs, and when it does, it often is fatal.

Both basal and squamous cell cancers are found mainly on areas of the skin exposed to the sun—the head, face, neck, hands, and arms. However, skin cancer can occur anywhere. Changes in the skin are not sure signs of cancer; however, it's important to see a doctor if any symptom lasts longer than two weeks. **Don't wait for the area to hurt—skin cancers seldom cause pain.**

All skin cancers could be cured if they were discovered and brought to a doctor's attention before they had a chance to spread. Therefore, you should check your skin regularly. The most common warning sign of skin cancer is a change on the skin, especially a new growth or a sore that doesn't heal. Skin cancers don't all look the same. For example, skin cancer can start as a small, smooth, shiny, pale, or waxy lump. Or it can appear as a firm red lump. Sometimes, the lump bleeds or develops a crust. Skin cancer also can start as a flat, red spot that is rough, dry, or scaly.

In treating skin cancer, the doctor's main goal is to remove or destroy cancer completely, leaving as small scar as possible. To plan the best treatment for each person, the doctor considers the type of skin cancer, its location and size, and the person's general health and medical history. Treatment for skin cancer usually involves some type of surgery. In some cases, radiation therapy or chemotherapy (anticancer drugs) or a combination of these treatments may be necessary.

Age Spots

Age spots, or *"liver spots"* as they're often called, have nothing to do with the liver. Rather, these flat, brown spots are caused by years of sun exposure. They are bigger than freckles and appear in fair-skinned people on sun-exposed areas such as the face, hands, arms, back, and feet. The medical name for them is solar lentigo. They may be accompanied by wrinkling, dryness, thinning of the skin, and rough spots.

A number of treatments are available, including skin-lightening, or "fade" creams; cryotherapy (freezing); and laser therapy. Tretinoin cream is approved for reducing the appearance of darkened spots. A sunscreen or sun block should be used to prevent further damage.

Shingles

Shingles is an outbreak of a rash or blisters on the skin that may cause severe pain. Shingles is caused by the varicella-zoster virus, the same virus that causes chickenpox. After an attack of chickenpox, the virus lies silent in the nerve tissue. Years later, the virus can reappear in the form of shingles. Although it is most common in people over age 50, anyone who has had chickenpox can develop shingles. It also is common in people with weakened immune systems due to HIV infection, chemotherapy or radiation treatment, transplant operations, and stress.

Early signs of shingles include burning or shooting pain and tingling or itching, generally on one side of the body or face. A rash appears as a band or patch of raised dots on the side of the trunk or face. The rash develops into small, fluid-filled blisters, which begin to dry out and crust over within several days. When the rash is at its peak, symptoms can range from mild itching to intense pain. Most people with shingles have only one bout with the disease in their lifetime. However, those with impaired immune systems—for example, people with AIDS or cancer—may suffer repeated episodes.

If you suspect you have shingles, see a doctor right away. The severity and duration of an attack of shingles can be reduced significantly by immediate treatment with antiviral drugs. These drugs also may help prevent the painful aftereffects of shingles known as postherpetic neuralgia. The National Institute of Allergy and Infectious Diseases has tested a shingles vaccine similar to the

SKIN CARE AND AGING

one used to immunize against chickenpox. Scientists hope that a vaccine to prevent shingles will be available in the future.

Bruising

Many older people notice an increased number of bruises, especially on their arms and legs. The skin becomes thinner with age and sun damage. Loss of fat and connective tissue weakens the support around blood vessels, making them more susceptible to injury. The skin bruises and tears more easily and takes longer to heal.

Sometimes bruising is caused by medications or illness. If bruising occurs in areas always covered by clothing, see a doctor.

Keep Your Skin Healthy

The best way to keep your skin healthy is to avoid sun exposure.

Stay out of the sun. Avoid the sun between 10 a.m. and 3 p.m. This is when the sun's UV rays are strongest. Don't be fooled by cloudy skies. Harmful rays pass through clouds. UV radiation also can pass through water, so don't assume you're safe if you're in the water and feeling cool.

Use sunscreen. Sunscreens are rated in strength according to a sun protection factor (SPF), which ranges from 2 to 30 or higher. A higher number means longer protection. Buy products with an SPF number of 15 or higher. Also look for products whose label says: broad spectrum (meaning they protect against both types of harmful sun rays—UVA and UVB) and water resistant (meaning they stay on your skin longer, even if you get wet or sweat a lot). Remember to reapply the lotion as needed.

Wear protective clothing. A hat with a wide brim shades your neck, ears, eyes, and head. Look for sunglasses with a label saying the glasses block 99 to 100% of the sun's rays. Wear loose, lightweight, long-sleeved shirts and long pants or long skirts when in the sun.

Avoid artificial tanning. Don't use sunlamps and tanning beds, as well as tanning pills and tanning makeup. Tanning pills have a color additive that turns your skin orange after you take them. The FDA has approved this color additive for coloring foods but not for tanning the skin. The large amount of color additive in tanning pills may be harmful. Tanning make-up products are not suntan lotions and will not protect your skin from the sun.

Check your skin often. Look for changes in the size, shape, color, or feel of birthmarks, moles, and spots. If you find any changes that worry you, see a doctor. The American Academy of Dermatology suggests that older, fair-skinned people have a yearly skin check by a doctor as part of a regular physical exam.

For More Information

The organizations listed below offer more information about some of the topics mentioned in this fact sheet:

National Institute of Arthritis and Musculoskeletal and Skin Diseases Clearinghouse
877-226-4267 (toll-free)
301-495-4484
www.niams.nih.gov

National Cancer Institute
800-422-6237 (toll-free)
www.cancer.gov

Food and Drug Administration
888-463-6332 (toll-free)
www.fda.gov

The American Academy of Dermatology
888-462-3376 (toll-free)
www.aad.org

For more information about health and aging, contact:

National Institute on Aging Information Center
P.O. Box 8057
Gaithersburg, MD 20898-8057
800-222-2225 (toll-free)
800-222-4225 (TTY/toll-free)

- To order publications (in English or Spanish) online, visit *www.niapublications.org*.
- The National Institute on Aging website is *www.nia.nih.gov*.

- Visit NIHSeniorHealth.gov (*www.nihseniorhealth.gov*), a senior-friendly website from the National Institute on Aging and the National Library of Medicine. This simple-to-use website features popular health topics for older adults. It has large type and a "talking" function that reads the text out loud.

October 2000

Smoking: It's Never Too Late to Stop

> "I've smoked two packs of cigarettes a day for 40 years—what's the use of quitting now?"

If you quit smoking, you are likely to add years to your life, breathe more easily, and have more energy. You will have extra money for spending or saving, and food will taste better. When you quit smoking, you join over a million people who stop smoking each year. Whether you are young or old, you will also:

- Have less chance of cancer, heart attack, and lung disease,
- Have better blood circulation,
- Have no odor of smoke in your clothes and hair,
- Set a healthy example for children and grandchildren,
- Have a more sensitive sense of smell,
- Have a better sense of taste, and
- Have healthier family members, particularly children and grandchildren.

What Smoking Does

Cigarette smoke damages your lungs and airways. Air passages swell and, over time, you will have more and more trouble clearing mucus from your air passages. This can cause a cough that won't go away. Sometimes this leads to a lung disease called chronic bronchitis. If you keep smoking, normal breathing may become harder and harder as emphysema develops. In emphysema, your lung tissue is destroyed, making it very hard to get enough oxygen.

Smoking can shorten your life. It brings an early death to more than 400,000 people in the United States each year. Lifelong smokers have a 1 in 2 chance of dying from a smoking-related disease. Smoking cuts years off the end of your life. Smoking makes millions of Americans sick by causing:

- *Heart Disease.* If you have high blood pressure or high cholesterol (a fatty substance in the blood) and also smoke, you increase your chance of having a heart attack. Quitting will greatly lower your risk of heart disease.
- *Cancer.* Smoking can cause cancer of the lungs, mouth, larynx (voice box), esophagus, stomach, liver, pancreas, kidney, bladder, and cervix. Your chance of getting cancer gets greater the more cigarettes you smoke each day and the more years you smoke.
- *Respiratory Problems.* If you smoke, you are more likely than a nonsmoker

to get the flu (influenza), pneumonia, or other infections that can interfere with your breathing. These can be very dangerous, especially for older people.

- *Osteoporosis.* If you are an older woman who smokes, your chance of developing osteoporosis is greater. Women who are past menopause tend to lose bone strength and sometimes develop this bone-weakening disorder. Bones weakened by osteoporosis break more easily. Also, women smokers tend to begin menopause sooner than the average woman does, putting them at risk at an earlier age.

Good News About Quitting

As soon as you stop smoking, your lungs, heart, and circulatory system (the arteries and veins that blood flows through) start getting better.

- Your chance of heart attack, stroke, and other circulatory diseases begins to drop within the first year after you quit.
- Within one year of quitting you are almost half as likely to develop heart disease as you were before.
- The flow of blood to your hands and feet gets stronger.
- Your breathing becomes easier within a few months after your last cigarette.
- Your chance of getting cancer from smoking also begins to shrink. The sooner you quit, the greater the benefit to your health. Within 10 to 15 years after quitting, your risk of cancer may be almost as low as that of a nonsmoker.

Worried About Putting on Pounds?

You may be worried about gaining weight if you stop smoking. Don't be. Many people who stop smoking gain little or no weight. But, even if you add a few pounds, you will be healthier than if you continued smoking.

Nicotine Is a Drug

Nicotine is a drug-like chemical in cigarette smoke. It is the main reason tobacco products are addictive. At first, when you smoke, nicotine makes you feel good. This might make you want to smoke more. Soon, your body starts to need more nicotine in order to feel good. Then you smoke even more to keep getting that pleasurable feeling.

The first few weeks after quitting are the hardest. Some people who give up smoking have withdrawal symptoms. You may become grumpy, hungry, or tired. You may have headaches, feel depressed, or have problems sleeping or concentrating. Some people have no withdrawal symptoms at all.

Breaking the Addiction

Smoking is a strong addiction for both your body and mind. That is why it is so hard to stop. But, people do succeed. Since 1965 over 40 million Americans who used to smoke have quit. There is help. You can:

- Read self-help literature,
- Use individual or group counseling,
- Join a support group,
- Ask a friend to quit with you,
- Take medicine to help with nicotine withdrawal, or
- Use nicotine replacement therapy.

Each person is different. Find what works best for you. Sometimes combining several methods is the answer. Some people can stop on their own. Others—maybe you—need help from doctors, clinics, or organized groups.

The first step is to make a firm decision to quit. Then, choose a date to stop smoking, and pick one or more methods for quitting. Before you stop, try changing your smoking habits. For example, if you smoke a cigarette after each meal, wait a while at first. Perhaps you smoke while reading the newspaper. Try to chew gum instead. Then, when you do stop smoking, habits such as these may be easier to stop.

When you quit, you may need special help to cope with your body's desire for nicotine. Nicotine replacement therapy can help some smokers control withdrawal symptoms as they quit. You can buy some nicotine replacement products over-the-counter. Check with your doctor first to see if one is a good choice for you. He or she might recommend one of the over-the-counter forms:

- *Nicotine chewing gum,*
- *Nicotine patch, or*
- *Nicotine lozenge.*

But, these require a doctor's prescription:

- *Nicotine nasal spray or*
- *Nicotine inhaler*

These give nicotine to the body without the harmful substances found in tobacco smoke. They reduce withdrawal symptoms. This makes it easier for you to overcome your addiction to tobacco. Also, this dose of nicotine is less than that from a cigarette and is tapered off during the treatment period.

There is a drug to help you handle your cravings. Known as bupropion hydrochloride, it does not contain nicotine and must be prescribed by your doctor. The most common side effects are dry mouth and sleep problems.

Cigars, Pipes, Chewing Tobacco, and Snuff Are Not Safe

Some people think smokeless tobacco (chewing tobacco and snuff), pipes, and cigars are safe. They are not. Using smokeless tobacco can cause cancer of the mouth, pre-cancerous lesions known as oral leukoplakia, nicotine addiction, and possibly cancer of the larynx and esophagus, as well as gum problems. Pipe and cigar smokers may develop cancer of the mouth, lip, larynx, pharynx, esophagus, and bladder. Those who inhale are also at increased risk of getting lung cancer.

Secondhand Smoke

If you are around someone who smokes, you could be exposed to secondhand smoke from his or her cigarette, pipe, or cigar. We now know that secondhand smoke can make nonsmokers sick. Adults who don't smoke but live or work with smokers are more likely to develop lung cancer than other nonsmokers. It has also been linked to heart disease in nonsmokers.

Secondhand smoke is very dangerous for someone with asthma, other lung conditions, or heart disease. It may cause bronchitis, pneumonia, an asthma attack, or inner ear infections in babies and young children. It may be associated with SIDS (sudden infant death syndrome). These problems are just some good reasons for a parent or grandparent to think about quitting smoking. Everyone should try not to smoke indoors around others of any age.

Where to Get Help

Organizations, doctors, and clinics offering stop-smoking programs are listed in telephone books under headings such as "Smokers' Treatment and Information Centers."

For More Information

Further information can be obtained from organizations such as the following:

These three organizations have many local chapters which can be found in a local telephone directory.

American Cancer Society
1599 Clifton Road, NE
Atlanta, GA 30329
800-227-2345 (toll-free)
www.cancer.org

American Heart Association
7272 Greenville Avenue
Dallas, TX 75231
800-242-8721 (toll-free)
www.americanheart.org

American Lung Association
61 Broadway, Sixth Floor
New York, NY 10006
800-586-4872 (toll-free)
www.lungusa.org

Several government agencies also have information on the dangers of smoking.

Office on Smoking and Health Centers for Disease Control and Prevention
1600 Clifton Road, NE
Atlanta, GA 30333
800-311-3435 (toll-free)
www.cdc.gov/tobacco

National Cancer Institute
Cancer Information Service
6116 Executive Boulevard
Suite 3035A
Rockville, MD 20852
800-422-6237 (toll-free)
800-332-8615 (TTY/toll-free)
www.cancer.gov

Smokefree.gov
800-784-8669 (toll-free)
www.smokefree.gov

National Heart, Lung, and Blood Institute
Health Information Center
P.O. Box 30105
Bethesda, MD 20824-0105
301-592-8573
240-629-3255
www.nhlbi.nih.gov

National Library of Medicine MedlinePlus
www.medlineplus.gov

- In Health Topics, go to:
  "Secondhand Smoke"
  "Smoking"
  "Smoking Cessation"
  "Smokeless Tobacco"

For more information about health and aging, contact:

National Institute on Aging Information Center
P.O. Box 8057
Gaithersburg, MD 20898-8057
800-222-2225 (toll-free)
800-222-4225 (TTY/toll-free)

- To order publications (in English or Spanish) online, visit www.niapublications.org.

- The National Institute on Aging website is www.nia.nih.gov.

- Visit NIHSeniorHealth.gov (www.nihseniorhealth.gov), a senior-friendly website from the National Institute on Aging and the National Library of Medicine. This simple-to-use website features popular health topics for older adults, including one on lung cancer. It has large type and a "talking" function that reads the text out loud.

July 2004

Taking Care of Your Teeth and Mouth

No matter what your age, you need to take care of your teeth and mouth. When your mouth is healthy, you can easily eat the foods you need for good nutrition. Smiling, talking, and laughing with others also are easier when your mouth is healthy.

Tooth Decay (Cavities)

Teeth are meant to last a lifetime. By taking good care of your teeth and gums, you can protect them for years to come. Tooth decay is not just a problem for children. It can happen as long as you have natural teeth in your mouth.

Tooth decay ruins the enamel that covers and protects your teeth. When you don't take good care of your mouth, bacteria can cling to your teeth and form a sticky, colorless film called dental plaque. This plaque can lead to tooth decay and cavities. Gum disease can also cause your teeth to decay.

Fluoride is just as helpful for adults as it is for children. Using a fluoride toothpaste and mouth rinse can help protect your teeth. If you have a problem with cavities, your dentist or dental hygienist may give you a fluoride treatment during the office visit. The dentist also may prescribe a fluoride gel or mouth rinse for you to use at home.

Gum Diseases

Gum diseases (sometimes called *periodontal* or *gingival diseases*) are infections that harm the gum and bone that hold teeth in place. When plaque stays on your teeth too long, it forms a hard, harmful covering, called tartar, that brushing doesn't clean. The longer the plaque and tartar stay on your teeth, the more damage they cause. Your gums may become red, swollen, and bleed easily. This is called *gingivitis*.

If gingivitis is not treated, over time it can make your gums pull away from your teeth and form pockets that can get infected. This is called periodontitis. If not treated, this infection can ruin the bones, gums, and tissue that support your teeth. In time, it can cause loose teeth that your dentist may have to remove.

Here's how you can prevent gum disease:

- Brush your teeth twice a day (with a fluoride toothpaste).
- Floss once a day.
- Make regular visits to your dentist for a checkup and cleaning.
- Eat a well-balanced diet.
- Don't use tobacco products.

Cleaning Your Teeth and Gums

Knowing how to brush and floss the right way is a big part of good oral health.

Here's how: every day gently brush your teeth on all sides with a soft-bristle brush and fluoride toothpaste. Small round motions and short back-and-forth strokes work best. Take the time to brush carefully and gently along the gum line. Lightly brushing your tongue also helps.

Along with brushing, clean around your teeth with dental floss to keep your gums healthy.

Careful flossing will remove plaque and leftover food that a toothbrush can't reach. Rinse after you floss.

If brushing or flossing causes your gums to bleed or hurt your mouth, see your dentist.

Your dentist also may prescribe a bacteria-fighting mouth rinse to help control plaque and swollen gums. Use the mouth rinse in addition to careful daily brushing and flossing.

Some people with arthritis or other conditions that limit motion may find it hard to hold a toothbrush. It may help to attach the toothbrush handle to your hand with a wide elastic band. Some people make the handle bigger by taping it to a sponge or Styrofoam ball. People with limited shoulder movement may find brushing easier if they attach a long piece of wood or plastic to the handle. Electric toothbrushes can be helpful.

Dentures

Dentures (sometimes called false teeth) may feel strange at first. When you are learning to eat with them, it may be easier if you:

- Start with soft non-sticky food,
- Cut your food into small pieces, and
- Chew slowly using both sides of your mouth.

Dentures may make your mouth less sensitive to hot foods and liquids. They also may make it harder for you to notice harmful objects such as bones, so be

How To Floss

Step 1

Hold floss as shown.

Step 2

Use floss between upper teeth.

Step 3

Use floss between lower teeth.

careful. During the first few weeks you have dentures, your dentist may want to see you often to make sure they fit. Over time, your mouth changes and your dentures may need to be replaced or adjusted. Be sure to let your dentist handle these adjustments.

Keep your dentures clean and free from food that can cause stains, bad breath, or swollen gums. Once a day, brush all surfaces with a denture care product. When you go to sleep, take your dentures out of your mouth and put them in water or a denture cleansing liquid.

Take care of partial dentures the same way. Because bacteria can collect under the clasps (clips) that hold partial dentures, be sure to carefully clean that area.

Dental Implants

Dental implants are small metal pieces placed in the jaw to hold false teeth or partial dentures in place. They are not for everyone. You need a complete dental and medical checkup to find out if implants are right for you. Your gums must be healthy and your jawbone able to support the implants. Talk to your dentist to find out if you should think about dental implants.

Dry Mouth

Doctors used to think that dry mouth (xerostomia) was a normal part of aging. They now know that's not true. Older, healthy adults shouldn't have a problem with saliva.

Dry mouth happens when salivary glands don't work properly. This can make it hard to eat, swallow, taste, and even speak. Dry mouth also can add to the risk of tooth decay and infection. You can get dry mouth from many diseases or medical treatments, such as head and neck radiation therapy. Many common medicines also can cause dry mouth.

If you think you have dry mouth, talk with your dentist or doctor to find out why. If your dry mouth is caused by a medicine you take, your doctor might change your medicine or dosage.

To prevent the dryness, drink extra water. Cut back on sugary snacks, drinks that have caffeine or alcohol, and tobacco. Your dentist or doctor also might suggest that you keep your mouth wet by using artificial saliva, which you can get from most drug stores. Some people benefit from sucking hard candy.

Oral Cancer

Oral cancer most often occurs in people over age 40. It's important to catch oral cancer early, because treatment works best before the disease has spread. Pain often is not an early symptom of the disease.

A dental checkup is a good time for your dentist to look for early signs of oral cancer. Even if you have lost all your natural teeth, you should still see your dentist for regular oral cancer exams. See your dentist or doctor if you have trouble with swelling, numbness, sores, or lumps in your mouth, or if it becomes hard for you to chew, swallow, or move your jaw or tongue. These problems could be signs of oral cancer.

Here's how you can lower your risk of getting oral cancer: don't smoke; don't use snuff or chew tobacco; if you drink alcohol, do so in moderation; use lip cream with sunscreen; and eat lots of fruits and vegetables.

For More Information

If you have other questions about your teeth and oral health, contact:

National Institute of Dental and Craniofacial Research (NIDCR)
Building 45, Room 4AS19
45 Center Drive MSC 6400
Bethesda, MD 20892-6400
301-496-4261
www.nidcr.nih.gov

The American Dental Association (ADA) provides information about oral health topics.

American Dental Association (ADA)
211 East Chicago Avenue
Chicago, IL 60611
800-621-8099 (toll-free)
www.ada.org

For more information about health and aging, contact:

National Institute on Aging Information Center
P.O. Box 8057
Gaithersburg, MD 20898-8057
800-222-2225 (toll-free)
800-222-4225 (TTY/toll-free)

- To order publications (in English or Spanish) online, visit www.niapublications.org.
- The National Institute on Aging website is www.nia.nih.gov.
- Visit NIHSeniorHealth.gov (www.nihseniorhealth.gov), a senior-friendly website from the National Institute on Aging and the National Library of Medicine. This simple-to-use website features popular health topics for older adults. It has large type and a "talking" function that reads the text out loud.

January 2002

What to Do About Flu

Each winter, millions of people suffer from the flu, a highly contagious infection. It spreads easily from person to person mainly when an infected person coughs or sneezes. Flu—the short name for influenza—is caused by viruses that infect the nose, throat, and lungs. It usually is a mild disease in healthy children, young adults, and middle-aged people. However, flu can be life threatening in older adults and in people of any age who have chronic illnesses such as diabetes or heart, lung, or kidney diseases.

Can Flu be Prevented?

A flu shot can greatly lower your chances of getting the flu. Much of the illness and death caused by flu can be prevented by a yearly flu shot.

The cost of the flu shot is covered by Medicare. Many private health insurance plans also pay for the flu shot. You can get a flu shot at your doctor's office. You also may be able to get a flu shot from your local health department or from other health care providers.

No vaccine gives complete protection, and the flu shot is no exception. In older people and those with certain chronic illnesses, the flu shot often is less effective in preventing flu than in reducing symptoms and the risk of serious illness and death. Studies have shown that the flu shot reduces hospitalization by about 70 percent and death by about 85 percent among older people who are not in nursing homes. Among nursing home residents, the flu shot reduces the risk of hospitalization by about 50 percent, the risk of pneumonia by about 60 percent, and the risk of death by 75 to 80%.

Who Should Get the Flu Shot?

According to the Federal Government's Centers for Disease Control and Prevention, the following people are at risk for serious illness from the flu and should get a flu shot every year:

- People 65 years of age and older,
- Residents of nursing homes and other long-term care facilities,
- Adults and children who have chronic heart or lung diseases,
- Adults and children with diabetes, kidney disease, or severe forms of anemia,
- Health care workers in contact with people in high-risk groups, and
- Caregivers or people who live with someone in a high-risk group.

When is the Best Time to Get the Flu Shot?

In the United States, flu season usually occurs from November until April. Most people get the flu between late December and early March. The best time to get your flu shot is between September and mid-November. It takes about 1 to 2 weeks after you get the shot to develop protection.

Call Your Doctor if You Have Any Signs of Flu and:

- Your fever lasts; you may have a more serious infection.

- You have breathing or heart problems or other serious health problems.

- You are taking drugs to fight cancer or other drugs that weaken your body's natural defenses against illness.

- You feel sick and don't seem to be getting better.

- You have a cough that begins to produce phlegm.

- You are worried about your health.

Does the Shot Cause Side Effects?

The flu shot does not cause side effects in most people. Fewer than one-third of those who get the shot have some soreness, redness, or swelling on the arm where the shot is given. These side effects, which can last up to two days, rarely interfere with a person's daily activities. About 5 to 10% of people have mild side effects such as headache or low-grade fever for about a day after vaccination.

The flu shot is made from killed flu viruses, which cannot cause the flu. With very rare exceptions, the danger from getting flu—and possibly pneumonia—is far greater than the danger from the side effects of the shot.

One of these rare exceptions is people who have a severe allergy to eggs. The viruses for flu vaccines are grown in eggs and may cause serious reactions in people who are severely allergic to eggs. People who have a severe allergy to eggs should not get the flu shot.

Why Do You Need a Flu Shot Every Year?

Preventing flu is hard because flu viruses change all the time. This year's flu virus usually is slightly different from last year's virus. Every year the flu shot is updated to include the most current flu virus strains. That's one reason why flu shots will protect you for only 1 year.

What Are the Symptoms of the Flu?

Flu can cause fever, chills, dry cough, sore throat, runny or stuffy nose, as well as headache, muscle aches, and often extreme fatigue. Although nausea, vomiting, and diarrhea can sometimes accompany the flu, especially in children, gastrointestinal symptoms rarely occur. The illness that people call "stomach flu" is not influenza.

It's easy to confuse a common cold with the flu. Overall, cold symptoms are milder and don't last as long as the flu.

How Serious is Flu?

Most people who get the flu recover completely in 1 to 2 weeks, but some people develop serious and possibly life-threatening complications. While your body is busy fighting off the flu, you may be less able to resist a second infection. Older people and people with chronic illnesses run the greatest risk of getting secondary infections, especially pneumonia. In an average year, flu leads to about 20,000 deaths nationwide and many more hospitalizations.

How is Flu Treated?

If you get the flu, rest in bed, drink plenty of fluids, and take medication such as aspirin or acetaminophen to relieve fever and discomfort.

Antibiotics are not effective against flu viruses. However, four drugs have been approved to treat people who get the flu:

- Amantadine (Symmetrel),
- Rimantadine (Flumadine),
- Zanamivir (Relenza), and
- Oseltamivir (Tamiflu).

When taken within 48 hours after the onset of illness, these drugs reduce the duration of fever and other symptoms. These drugs are only available by prescription.

Facts About Flu

- **The flu can be very dangerous for people 65 and older.**
- **The flu can be prevented.**
- **A flu shot is necessary each fall for people in high-risk groups.**
- **The flu shot is covered by Medicare.**
- **The flu shot is safe. It can't cause the flu.**
- **The flu shot and the pneumococcal vaccine can be given at the same time.**

For More Information

To learn more about flu and other adult immunizations, contact the following groups:

National Institute of Allergy and Infectious Diseases
301-496-5717
www.niaid.nih.gov

Centers for Disease Control and Prevention
National Immunization Information Hotline
800-232-4636 (toll-free)
www.cdc.gov

Food and Drug Administration
888-463-6332 (toll-free)
www.fda.gov

American Lung Association
800-586-4872 (toll-free)
www.lungusa.org

National Coalition for Adult Immunization
4733 Bethesda Avenue
Suite 750
Bethesda, MD 20814
301-656-0003
www.nfid.org/ncai

For more information about health and aging, contact:

National Institute on Aging Information Center
P.O. Box 8057
Gaithersburg, MD 20898-8057
800-222-2225 (toll-free)
800-222-4225 (TTY/toll-free)

- To order publications (in English or Spanish) online, visit www.niapublications.org.

- The National Institute on Aging website is www.nia.nih.gov.

- Visit NIHSeniorHealth.gov (www.nihseniorhealth.gov), a senior-friendly website from the National Institute on Aging and the National Library of Medicine. This simple-to-use website features popular health topics for older adults. It has large type and a "talking" function that reads the text out loud.

February 2000

Getting Good Health Care

What to remember when you need medical help

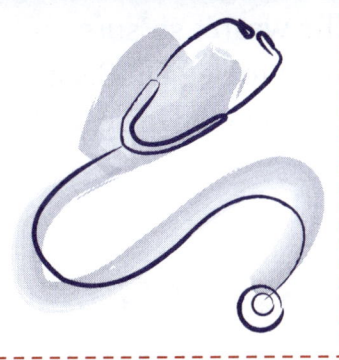

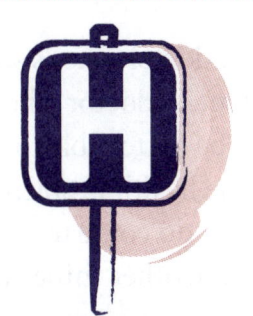

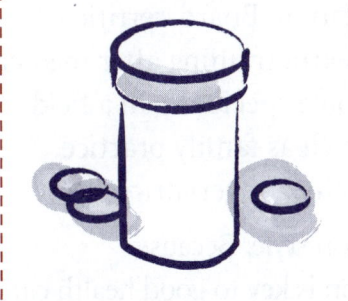

- 134 **Choosing a Doctor**
- 139 **Considering Surgery?**
- 142 **Health Quackery: Spotting Health Scams**
- 145 **Hospital Hints**
- 150 **Medicines: Use Them Safely**
- 153 **Online Health Information: Can You Trust It?**

Choosing a Doctor

Mrs. Wiley had a big surprise the other day when she called her doctor to make an appointment. The receptionist told her that Dr. Horowitz was retiring at the end of the year. After all this time—after decades of flu, bladder infections, and that nasty broken wrist; after helping her through the menopause—now this desertion! Mrs. Wiley didn't know what she would do to try and find a new doctor.

Uncle Willy was grumbling to his nephew Matt. This new managed health insurance plan seemed like a good idea at first, but now he wasn't so sure. What's a primary care doctor anyway? Can't he just continue to see Dr. Bissell for his arthritis? Matt sighed, wondering how he was going to help Uncle Willy find a whole new set of doctors.

Stories like these are becoming all too common. Finding good medical care can be tricky at any age, but for older people this task may be even tougher. Yet, it is important to have a primary care doctor who knows you and all of your health problems. Even if you see other doctors for certain health conditions, for example, a heart specialist (cardiologist) for heart disease, your primary care doctor is needed to work with those specialists and coordinate all of your health care.

Choosing a doctor is one of the most important decisions anyone can make. The best time to make that decision is while you are still healthy and have time to really think about all your choices. If you have no doctor or are thinking of changing doctors, the following ideas may help you find a doctor who is right for you.

What Should You Look for in a Doctor?

Of course you want a doctor who is well trained and competent. A doctor who knows you well may be better able to help you prevent some health problems and manage those that do come up. In choosing a doctor some other things to think about are:

- Board certification. Board-certified doctors have extra training after medical school to become specialists in a field of medicine such as family practice, internal medicine, or geriatrics.
- Communication style. Because communication is key to good health care, you want a doctor who will listen carefully to your concerns, answer your questions, and explain things clearly and fully.
- Type of health insurance—does the doctor accept Medicare predetermined payments?

- The location of the doctor's office—will it be easy for you to get there?
- Where patients get lab work done—in the doctor's office or somewhere else?
- Whether the office staff will process your medical insurance claims for you.
- Which hospital the doctor uses to treat patients.
- Whether the doctor works with a group of other doctors. If so, who are the others, and what are their specialties?
- Who covers for the doctor if he/she is out of town or not available?
- Whether, with your permission, the doctor will share information with a family member.
- Which languages the doctor speaks.

A good first step is to make a list of the things that matter most to you. Then, go back over your list, and rank them in order of importance.

What Type of Doctor?

For your primary care doctor, you might want a general or family practitioner, an internist, or a geriatrician.

- General practitioners provide health care for a wide range of medical problems. They do not focus on any one area of medicine.
- Family practitioners are similar to general practitioners, with extra training to focus on health care for all family members, regardless of age.
- An internist is a doctor for adults. Some internists take additional training to become specialists. For example, cardiologists are internists who specialize in diseases of the heart.
- Geriatricians specialize in the care of older adults. A geriatrician is trained in family practice or internal medicine, but has additional training in caring for older people.

How Does Managed Care Affect Your Choice of Doctors?

Most people age 65 and older are eligible for Medicare hospital insurance (Part A). They also can enroll in Medicare medical insurance (Part B) for a monthly fee. Medicare medical insurance helps pay for visits to the doctor. It also covers many other medical services and supplies not covered by Medicare's Part A.

Many older people use Medicare's original fee-for-service health insurance program. Under this program, you may see any doctor or health care provider you choose. You usually pay Medicare's deductible and co-insurance, along with any other charges not covered by Medicare. Medicare pays the rest. Under this plan, you handle bills and payments.

Another option is a Medicare managed care plan. When you enroll in a managed care plan, you choose your doctor from a list of primary care doctors who are part

CHOOSING A DOCTOR **135**

of that plan's network. Your primary care doctor then coordinates all of your health care needs. If you do not choose a primary care doctor, the managed care plan will assign one to you.

In some managed care plans, you can see a doctor outside the network, but it will cost you more money. Also, you may have to pay a co-payment for some services and visits.

Today, there are many different kinds of managed care plans. Their benefits, costs, and rules vary. Be sure to compare each plan and consider the type of insurance (fee-for-service vs. managed care) that is best for you.

For information about Medicare benefits, call the Social Security Administration office listed in your phone book. Or call the toll-free Medicare hotline at 800-MEDICARE (800-633-4227). Information about Medicare eligibility, enrollment, insurance plans, and more is also available online at *www.medicare.gov*.

Finding a New Doctor

Once you have a sense of what you want in a doctor, ask people you know about doctors they use and like. Friends, coworkers, and other health professionals may be helpful. You can make it easy for them to tell you about the doctors they like by asking questions, such as, "What do you like about Dr. Smith?"

A doctor whose name comes up often might be a strong possibility as a choice. It may help to have several names to choose from in case the doctor you select is not taking new patients or does not take part in your health insurance plan.

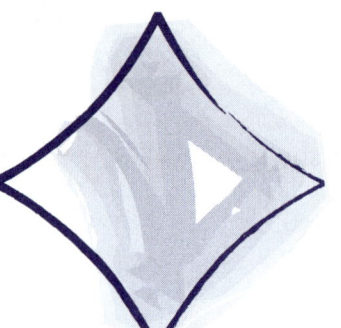

If you belong to a managed care plan, you can get a list of doctors from the plan's membership services office. Your choices will be limited to those doctors who are part of the plan.

If you need more help finding names of doctors, contact your hospital of choice, local medical society, local physician referral services, nearby medical schools, or university medical centers in your area.

How Do You Make an Informed Choice?

Once you have chosen two or three doctors, call their offices. The office staff can give you information about the doctor's education and training. They also can tell you about office policies, standard insurance the office takes, payment methods, and the doctor's hospital admitting privileges.

You may want to make an appointment just to talk with a doctor before deciding on a final choice. Make sure that she or he knows that you are trying to decide on a doctor. You likely will be charged for such a visit; your insurance company may not pay for it.

Make a list of questions you want to ask the doctor. For example:

- What age groups make up most of your practice?
- How do you manage patients with lots of health problems? Do you usually treat everything, do you refer patients, or are there some problems older people just have to live with?
- What do you think are the most important preventive care issues for older adults? How do you manage them?
- What's the best way for me to prepare for an office visit with you? For example, should I bring my questions in writing?
- Would you provide your instructions in writing for me?
- May I bring a family member (spouse, daughter, or son) to my office visits with you?
- If I give you permission, are you comfortable talking with my family about my condition?
- How do you involve your patients in health care decisions?
- Do you see many patients with the same chronic health problem that I have (for example, diabetes)?

After the meeting, ask yourself if you felt comfortable and confident with this doctor. Were you at ease asking questions? Did the doctor clearly answer your questions? If you are not sure, schedule a visit with one of the other doctors on your list.

The First Appointment

After choosing a doctor, make your first medical appointment. During this visit, the doctor will probably take a medical history and ask questions about your health. There may be questions about the health of your family members as well. The doctor also will examine you. Be sure to bring your past medical records (or have them sent). Also bring all of the medicines you take with you to show the doctor. Include both prescription and over-the counter drugs, even vitamins, supplements, and eye drops. Make a list of any drug allergies or serious drug reactions you've had. During this visit take time to ask any questions you may still have about the doctor and the practice.

Once you have found a doctor you like, your job is not finished. A good doctor-patient relationship is a partnership. Both you and your doctor need to work together to solve your medical problems and maintain your good health. Finding a medical practice that is well suited to your needs is an important first step. Good communication with the doctor and the office staff is the key.

CHOOSING A DOCTOR **137**

For More Information

The following organizations may be able to help you find a doctor:

American Geriatrics Society (AGS)
The Empire State Building
350 Fifth Avenue, Suite 801
New York, NY 10118
www.americangeriatrics.org

- AGS Referral Phone Line: 800-247-4779 (toll-free)

American College of Physicians-American Society of Internal Medicine
190 North Independence Mall West
Philadelphia, PA 19106-1572
800-523-1546 (toll-free)
www.acponline.org

American Academy of Family Physicians
11400 Tomahawk Creek Parkway
Leawood, KS 66211
800-274-2237 (toll-free)
www.aafp.org

American Medical Association
515 North State Street
Chicago, IL 60610
800-621-8335 (toll-free)
www.ama-assn.org

American Osteopathic Association
142 East Ontario Street
Chicago, IL 60611
800-621-1773 (toll-free)
www.osteopathic.org

Centers for Medicare & Medicaid Services
7500 Security Boulevard
Baltimore MD 21244-1850
800-633-4227 (toll-free)
www.medicare.gov

For more information about health and aging, contact:

National Institute on Aging Information Center
P.O. Box 8057
Gaithersburg, MD 20898-8057
800-222-2225 (toll-free)
800-222-4225 (TTY/toll-free)

- To order publications (in English or Spanish) online, visit www.niapublications.org.

- The National Institute on Aging website is www.nia.nih.gov.

- Visit NIHSeniorHealth.gov (www.nihseniorhealth.gov), a senior-friendly website from the National Institute on Aging and the National Library of Medicine. This simple-to-use website features popular health topics for older adults. It has large type and a "talking" function that reads the text out loud.

September 2002

Considering Surgery?

Have you been told that you need to have surgery? If so, you are not alone. Millions of older Americans have surgery each year.

Most surgeries are not emergencies. You have time to find out as much as possible about the surgery, think the matter over, and review other options. You also have time to get a second opinion.

Questions to Ask

Deciding to have surgery can be difficult, but an informed decision may be easier to make once you know why surgery is necessary and whether there are other treatment choices. Your surgeon can help. Talk with your surgeon about your condition and the surgery recommended.

Don't hesitate to ask the surgeon any questions you might have. For example, do the benefits of surgery outweigh the risks?

Your surgeon should welcome your questions. If you don't understand something, ask the surgeon to explain it more clearly. The answers to the following questions will help you become informed and make the best decision.

- What surgery is recommended?
- Why do I need surgery?
- Can another treatment be tried instead of surgery?
- What if I don't have the surgery?
- How will the surgery affect my health and lifestyle?
- Are there any activities that I won't be able to do after surgery?
- How long will it take to recover?
- How much experience has the surgeon had doing this kind of surgery?
- Where will the surgery be done—in the hospital, the doctor's office, a special surgical center, or a day surgery unit of a hospital?
- What kind of anesthesia will be used? What are the side effects and risks of having anesthesia?
- Is there anything else I should know about this surgery?

Choosing a Surgeon

Your primary care doctor may recommend a surgeon to you. You also may want to identify another independent surgeon to get a second opinion.

One way to reduce the risk of surgery is to choose a surgeon who has been thoroughly trained to do the type of surgery you need and who has plenty of experience doing it. Be sure to ask about your surgeon's qualifications. For example, you may want to find out if your surgeon is certified by a surgical board that is approved by the American Board of Medical Specialties (such as the American Board of Orthopaedic Surgery, the American

Board of Colon and Rectal Surgery, or other national surgical board). Surgeons who are board certified have successfully completed training and passed exams for their specialty.

The letters "FACS" after a surgeon's name tell you that he or she is a Fellow of the American College of Surgeons. Fellows are almost always board-certified surgeons who have passed a test of their surgical training and skills; they also have shown their commitment to high standards of ethical conduct.

Don't hesitate to call the doctor's office and ask for this information. Your state or local medical society and the hospital where the surgeon operates also should be able to verify his or her training. Try to choose an experienced surgeon who operates regularly (several times a week) and who has treated a problem like yours before.

Getting a Second Opinion

Getting a second opinion from another surgeon is a good way to make sure that having surgery is the best choice for you. Many people are uneasy about seeking another opinion. They worry that they might offend their doctor. However, getting a second opinion is a common medical practice. Most doctors encourage it.

Getting a second opinion is a good way to get additional expert advice from another doctor who knows a lot about treating your particular medical problem. In addition, a second opinion can reassure you that your decision to have surgery is the right one.

Don't be afraid to tell your surgeon that you want another opinion and that you would like your medical records sent to the second doctor. This can save time, money, and possible discomfort since tests that you've already had may not need to be repeated if the second doctor has the results.

When getting another opinion, tell the second doctor your symptoms, the type of surgery that has been recommended, and the results of any tests you've already had. Ask the second doctor the same questions you asked the first one about the benefits and risks of surgery.

Medicare and many private health insurance companies will help pay for a second opinion. Most Medicaid programs also pay for a second opinion. If the second doctor agrees that surgery is needed, he or she usually will refer you back to the first doctor for the surgery.

If the second doctor disagrees with the first, you may feel you have enough information to decide what to do, you may wish to talk again with the first surgeon, or you may wish to see a third doctor. Your primary care doctor also may be able to help you decide what to do.

Informed Consent

Before having surgery, you'll be asked to give consent. It's important to discuss all of your concerns about your condition and the surgery with your surgeon before you sign this form. In most cases, your surgeon will volunteer a great deal of information, but don't hesitate to ask any questions you still have. Your doctor should be willing to take whatever time is necessary to make sure that you are fully informed.

Paying for Surgery

Before your surgery, ask about your surgeon's fees. Many surgeons volunteer this information; if yours doesn't, don't hesitate to ask. You can find out about hospital rates from the hospital business office. Your doctor should be able to tell you how long you can expect to be in the hospital. Today, many types of surgery can be performed without hospitalization. Your surgeon will be able to decide if that's possible in your case.

In addition to surgeons' fees and the costs of hospitalization, you also will be billed for the professional services of others involved in your care such as the anesthesiologist and medical consultants.

You may want to check your health insurance plan to see what portion of the costs you'll have to pay. You probably will need approval from your health insurance plan before surgery. If your insurance plan will not pay all of the anticipated costs and you cannot afford the difference, discuss this situation frankly with your surgeon.

Most people 65 and older have Medicare health insurance, which has two parts: Part A (hospital insurance) and Part B (medical insurance). Medicare Part A helps pay your hospital bill. It covers a semiprivate room, meals, general nursing, and other hospital services and supplies. It does not pay for private duty nursing, a television or telephone in your room, or a private room, unless medically necessary. For more information about Medicare coverage, call the toll-free helpline at 800-MEDICARE (800-633-4227).

For More Information

The organizations listed below offer more information about some of the topics mentioned in this fact sheet:

American College of Surgeons
633 North Saint Clair Street
Chicago, IL 60611-3211
800-621-4111 (toll-free)
312-202-5000
www.facs.org

American Society of Anesthesiologists
520 Northwest Highway
Park Ridge, IL 60068-2573
847-825-5586
www.asahq.org

For more information about health and aging, contact:

National Institute on Aging Information Center
P.O. Box 8057
Gaithersburg, MD 20898-8057
800-222-2225 (toll-free)
800-222-4225 (TTY/toll-free)

- To order publications (in English or Spanish) online, visit www.niapublications.org.
- The National Institute on Aging website is www.nia.nih.gov.

- Visit NIHSeniorHealth.gov (www.nihseniorhealth.gov), a senior-friendly website from the National Institute on Aging and the National Library of Medicine. This simple-to-use website features popular health topics for older adults. It has large type and a "talking" function that reads the text out loud.

February 2000

Health Quackery: Spotting Health Scams

You see the ads everywhere these days—"Smart Drugs for Long Life" or "Arthritis Aches and Pains Disappear Like Magic!" or even testimonials claiming, "This treatment cured my cancer in one week." It's easy to understand the appeal of these promises. But there is still plenty of truth to the old saying, "If it sounds too good to be true, it probably is!"

Quacks—people who sell unproven remedies—have been around for years. Today they have more ways than ever to peddle their wares. In addition to TV, radio, magazines, newspapers, infomercials, mail, and even word-of-mouth, they now can use the Internet—websites offer miracle cures; e-mails tell stories of overnight magic. Sadly, older people are often the target for such scams. In fact, a government study found that most victims of health care fraud are over age 65.

The problem is serious. Unproven remedies may be harmful. They may also waste money. And, sometimes, using these remedies keeps people from getting the medical treatment they need.

What Do Quacks Promise?

Unproven remedies promise false hope. Often they offer cures that are painless or quick. Why do people fall for these sales pitches? After all, at best these treatments are worthless. At worst, they are dangerous. One reason health care scams work is that they prey on people who are frightened or in pain. Living with a chronic health problem is hard. It's easy to see why people might fall for a false promise of a quick and painless cure.

You may see unproven remedies in products for:

Anti-Aging. Claims for pills or treatments that lead to eternal youth play on the great value our culture places on staying young. But, aging is normal. A product may smooth your wrinkles, but no treatments have yet been proven to slow the aging process. Eating a healthy diet, getting regular exercise, and not smoking are your best bets to help prevent some of the diseases that occur more often with age. In other words, making healthy lifestyle choices can increase your chances of aging well.

Arthritis Remedies. Unproven arthritis remedies can be easy to fall for because symptoms of arthritis tend to come and go. You may believe the remedy you are using is making you feel better when, in fact, it is just the normal ebb and flow of your symptoms. You may see claims that so-called treatments with herbs, oils, chemicals, special diets, radiation, and other products cured arthritis. This is highly unlikely. Individual testimonials alone do not guarantee that a product is effective. Instead, scientific studies proving that a treatment works are needed. While these products may not hurt you, they are costly and aren't likely to help much either. There is no cure for most forms of arthritis, but rest, exercise, heat, and drugs can help many people control their symptoms. If you are thinking about a new treatment, talk with your doctor first.

Cancer Cures. Quacks prey on people's fear of cancer. They promote treatments with no proven value—for example, a diet dangerously low in protein or drugs such as Laetrile. By using unproven methods, people with cancer may lose valuable time and the chance to receive a proven, effective treatment. This delay may lessen the chance for controlling or curing the disease.

Memory Aids. Many people worry about losing their memory as they age. They may wrongly believe false promises that unproven treatments can help them keep or improve their memory. So-called smart pills, removal of amalgam dental fillings, and brain retraining exercises are all examples of untested approaches that claim to help memory.

How Can You Protect Yourself From Health Scams?

Be wary. Question what you see or hear in ads or on the Internet. Newspapers, magazines, radio, and TV stations do not always check to make sure the claims in their ads are true. Find out about a product before you buy. Don't let a sales person force you to make a snap decision. Check with your doctor first.

Remember stories about the old snake oil salesman who traveled from town to town making claims for his fabulous product? Well, chances are today's quack is using the same sales tricks. Look for red flags in ads or promotional material that:

- Promise a quick or painless cure,
- Claim to be made from a special, secret, or ancient formula—often only available by mail or from one sponsor,
- Use testimonials or undocumented case histories from satisfied patients,
- Claim to be effective for a wide range of ailments,
- Claim to cure a disease (such as arthritis or cancer) that is not yet understood by medical science,
- Offer an additional "free" gift or a larger amount of the product as a "special promotion," or
- Require advance payment and claim limited availability of the product.

For More Information

If you have questions about a product, talk to your doctor or contact one of the organizations below. Get the facts about health products and protect yourself from health care hoaxes:

National Cancer Institute (NCI) Cancer Information Service (CIS)
800-422-6237 (toll-free)
800-332-8615 (TTY/toll-free)
www.cancer.gov

National Arthritis and Musculoskeletal and Skin Diseases Information Clearinghouse (NIAMS)
1 AMS Circle
Bethesda, MD 20892
877-226-4267 (toll-free)
301-565-2966 (TTY)
www.niams.nih.gov

Council of Better Business Bureaus (CBBB)
4200 Wilson Boulevard
8th Floor
Arlington, VA 22203
www.bbb.org

- Check the telephone book for the number of your local chapter.

Federal Trade Commission (FTC)
6th Street and Pennsylvania Avenue, NW
Room 421
Washington, DC 20580
877-382-4357 (toll-free)
800-326-2996 (TTY/toll-free)
www.ftc.gov

Food and Drug Administration (FDA)
5600 Fishers Lane
Rockville, MD 20857-0001
888-463-6332 (toll-free)
www.fda.gov

United States Postal Inspection Service (USPS)
Office of Investigation
Washington, DC 20206-2166
www.usps.com/postalinspectors/fraud/

- Check the telephone book for the number of your local postal inspector.

Quackwatch, Inc.
www.quackwatch.org

- Quackwatch, Inc, is a nonprofit corporation making information available to combat health-related frauds, myths, fads, and fallacies.

For more information about health and aging, contact:

National Institute on Aging Information Center
P.O. Box 8057
Gaithersburg, MD 20898-8057
800-222-2225 (toll-free)
800-222-4225 (TTY/toll-free)

- To order publications (in English or Spanish) online, visit www.niapublications.org.
- The National Institute on Aging website is www.nia.nih.gov.
- Visit NIHSeniorHealth.gov (www.nihseniorhealth.gov), a senior-friendly website from the National Institute on Aging and the National Library of Medicine. This simple-to-use website features popular health topics for older adults. It has large type and a "talking" function that reads the text out loud.

September 2002

Hospital Hints

Going to the hospital is somewhat like traveling to another country—the sights are unfamiliar and the people you meet there often speak a foreign language. No matter what the reason for the trip—whether it's an overnight visit for a few tests or a longer stay for medical treatment or major surgery—nearly everyone worries about entering the hospital. Learning more about hospitals and the people who work there may help make your hospital stay less stressful.

The following hints are meant for people who plan to enter the hospital by choice rather than for those who go to the hospital because of an emergency. (Information about emergency care is at the end of this *Age Page*.) Relatives and friends of patients who are admitted to the hospital also may find this information useful.

What to Bring

It's best to pack as little as you can. However, be sure to bring the following items:

- Nightclothes, bathrobe, and sturdy slippers (label all personal items),
- Comfortable clothes to wear home,
- A toothbrush, toothpaste, shampoo, comb and brush, deodorant, and razor,
- A list of your medicines, including prescription and over-the-counter drugs,
- Details of past illnesses, surgeries, and any allergies,
- Your health insurance card,
- A list of the names and telephone numbers (home and business) of family members to contact in an emergency, and
- Ten dollars or less for newspapers, magazines, or other items you may wish to buy in the hospital gift shop.

What to Leave Home

Leave jewelry (including wedding rings, earrings, and watches), credit cards, and checkbooks at home or have a family member or friend keep them for you. If you must bring valuables, ask if they can be kept in the hospital safe during your stay. In addition, leave electric razors, hair dryers, and curling irons at home.

Admission

Your first stop in the hospital will be the admitting office. Here you'll sign forms allowing the hospital staff to treat you and to release medical information to your insurance company. You also will be asked about advance directives (explained later in this *Age Page*).

Most people 65 and older have Medicare health insurance, which has two parts: Part A (hospital insurance) and Part B (medical insurance). Medicare Part A helps pay for care in hospitals, skilled nursing facilities, and hospices, as well as some home health care. It covers a semiprivate room, meals, general nursing, and other hospital services and supplies. It does not pay for private duty nursing, a television or telephone in your room, or a private room, unless medically necessary. For more information about Medicare coverage, call the toll-free helpline at 800-MEDICARE (800-633-4227).

If you don't have health insurance, an admissions counselor can advise you about other payment methods and sources of financial aid, such as the Hill-Burton program. Hill-Burton hospitals provide free or below-cost health care to people unable to pay. Eligibility for these free services is based on family size and income. For more information, call the Hill-Burton hotline at 800-638-0742; Maryland residents should call 800-492-0359.

Hospital Staff

Once you've filled out all the forms, you'll be taken to your room. You will then begin to meet the health professionals who will care for you while you're in the hospital.

Doctors are in charge of your overall care. You'll have an attending physician, who may be your primary doctor, a doctor on the hospital staff to whom you've been referred, or a specialist. In a teaching hospital (where doctors train), several doctors care for each patient. For example, the attending physician directs the house staff—medical students, residents (doctors who have recently graduated from medical school), and fellows (doctors who receive training in a special area of medicine or surgery after their residency training).

Nurses—registered nurses, nurse practitioners, licensed practical nurses, nurse's aides, and nursing students—provide many patient-care services. For example, nurses give medicines, check vital signs (blood pressure, temperature, and pulse), provide treatments, and teach patients to care for themselves. The head nurse coordinates nursing care for each patient on the unit (the floor or section of the hospital where your room is located).

Physical therapists teach patients how to build muscles, increase flexibility, and improve coordination. They may use exercise, heat, cold, or water therapy to help patients whose ability to move is limited.

Occupational therapists work with patients to restore, maintain, or increase their ability to perform daily tasks such as cooking, eating, bathing, and dressing.

Respiratory therapists prevent and treat breathing problems. For example, they teach patients exercises to help prevent lung infections after surgery.

Technicians perform a variety of tests such as x-rays and procedures such as taking blood.

Dietitians help plan specialized menus for patients and teach them how to plan a well-balanced diet.

Pharmacists know the chemical makeup and correct use of drugs. They prepare the medicines used in the hospital.

Social workers offer support to patients and their families. They can help patients and families learn about home care, social services, and support groups.

Discharge planners help patients arrange for health and home care needs after they go home from the hospital.

Geriatric Assessment

Some older people have many health problems that threaten their ability to live on their own after they leave the hospital. In some hospitals, a team that includes a doctor, nurse, and social worker addresses the special needs of older patients. This team also may include other specialists and therapists. The team performs a thorough exam, called a geriatric assessment, to learn about the patient's physical and mental health, family life, income, living arrangements, access to community services, and ability to perform daily tasks. The team diagnoses health problems and develops a plan to help older patients get the health care and social services they need.

Hospital Geography

Hospitals have many patient-care areas. For example, patients may be in a private (one-bed) or semiprivate (two-bed) room. The intensive care unit (also called the ICU) has special equipment and staff to care for very ill patients. The coronary care unit (CCU) gives intensive medical care to patients with severe heart disease. In both the ICU and CCU, visiting hours are strictly limited and usually only family members are allowed to see patients. Surgery is done in the operating room (OR). After an operation, patients spend time in the recovery room before going back to their own room.

In the emergency room (ER), trained staff treat life-threatening injuries or illnesses. Patients who are badly hurt or very sick are seen first. Because the ER is so busy, less seriously ill patients may have to wait before they are seen by an emergency medical technician, nurse, or doctor.

Safety Tips

Because you may feel weak or tired, please take a few extra safety steps while in the hospital:

- Use the call bell or button when you need help.
- Use the controls to lower your bed before getting in or out.
- Be careful not to trip over the wires and tubes that may be around the bed.
- Try to keep the things you need within easy reach.
- Take only prescribed medicines. If you bring your own medicines with you, tell your nurse or doctor. Don't take other drugs without your doctor's permission.
- Hold on to grab bars for support when getting in and out of the bathtub or shower.
- Use handrails on stairways and in hallways.

Questions

During your hospital stay, you'll probably have many questions about your care. Always feel free to ask your doctor these questions. Your doctor is there to help you get the care you need and to discuss your concerns. Your nurse or social worker also may be able to answer many of your questions or help you get the information you need.

You may find it useful to write down your questions as you think of them. For example, you may want to ask your doctor or nurse some or all of the following questions:

- What will this test tell you? Why is it needed, and when will you know the results?
- What treatment is needed, and how long will it last?
- What are the benefits and risks of treatment?
- When can I go home?
- When I go home, will I have to change my regular activities or my diet?
- How often will I need checkups?
- Is any other follow-up needed?

Patient Rights

You can decide in advance what medical treatments you want or don't want in the hospital in case you lose your ability to speak for yourself. You can do this by preparing something called an advance directive. In an advance directive, you tell people how to make medical decisions for you when you can't make them for yourself. You also can name someone else to make medical decisions for you. Two common advance directives are a living will and a durable power of attorney for health care.

In a living will, you write down the kind of medical care you want (or don't want) in case you are unable to make your own decisions. It's called a living will because it takes effect while you are still alive.

In a durable power of attorney for health care, you name someone else (a family member or friend, for example) to make medical decisions for you if you are unable to make them for yourself. You also can include instructions about any treatment you want to avoid.

If you have an advance directive, tell your family and make sure they know where it's located. Also, tell your doctor and make sure that the advance directive is part of your medical records. If you have a durable power of attorney for health care, give a copy to the person you've chosen to act on your behalf.

If you need help to prepare an advance directive or if you would like more information about them, contact your doctor or lawyer. You also can consult your State Attorney General's Office or State Office on Aging.

Discharge Planning

Before going home, you'll need discharge orders from your doctor and a release form from the hospital business office. Discharge planning before leaving the hospital can help you prepare for your health and home care needs after you go home. The discharge planner can help you arrange for a visiting nurse, hospital equipment, meals-on-wheels, or other services. The discharge planner also knows about senior centers, rehabilitation centers, nursing homes, and other long-term care services.

In Case of Emergency

In a medical emergency, every second counts! You may have severe pain, a bad injury, or sudden severe illness. In such a life-threatening emergency, seek medical help right away. In many areas, you can reach emergency help by calling 911 or the telephone operator. Be sure to tell the operator the type of emergency and your location.

When you need care for a sudden illness or injury that you don't think is an emergency, call your doctor or urgent care center. Often a visit to the emergency room (ER) isn't needed. If you do need to go to the ER, your doctor can make things easier for you by calling the hospital to let them know you are coming.

If there is time, try to take the following items with you to the ER:

- Your health insurance card or policy number,
- Your doctor's name and telephone number,
- A list of the medicines you take, including prescription and over-the-counter drugs, and
- The names and telephone numbers of close family members.

It's a good idea to write this information on a note card and carry it in your wallet or purse. If you have a medical problem such as epilepsy, diabetes, or allergies, you should wear an ID bracelet or carry an ID card to let rescue workers and hospital staff know about these hidden conditions.

If possible, ask a relative or friend to go to the hospital with you for support.

For More Information

The organizations listed below offer more information about some of the topics mentioned in this fact sheet:

The American Hospital Association provides information about hospitals and patient rights. Their address is:

American Hospital Association
One North Franklin
Chicago, IL 60606
312-422-3000
www.aha.org

For more information about health and aging, contact:

National Institute on Aging Information Center
P.O. Box 8057
Gaithersburg, MD 20898-8057
800-222-2225 (toll-free)
800-222-4225 (TTY/toll-free)

- To order publications (in English or Spanish) online, visit www.niapublications.org.
- The National Institute on Aging website is www.nia.nih.gov.

- Visit NIHSeniorHealth.gov (www.nihseniorhealth.gov), a senior-friendly website from the National Institute on Aging and the National Library of Medicine. This simple-to-use website features popular health topics for older adults. It has large type and a "talking" function that reads the text out loud.

February 2000

Medicines: Use Them Safely

People age 65 and older consume more prescription and over-the-counter (OTC) medicines than any other age group. Older people tend to have more long-term, chronic illnesses—such as arthritis, diabetes, high blood pressure and heart disease—than do younger people. Because they may have a number of diseases or disabilities at the same time, it is common for older people to take many different drugs.

Many older people owe their health in part to new and improved medicines and vaccines. But using medicines may be riskier for older adults, especially when several medicines are used at one time. Taking different medicines is not always easy to do right. It may be hard to remember what each medicine is for, how you should take it, and when you should take it. This is especially true of people with memory problems or dementia.

Medicines may act differently in older people than in younger people. This may be because of normal changes in the body that happen with age. For instance, as we get older, we lose water and lean tissue (mainly muscle) and we gain more fat tissue. This can make a difference in how long a drug stays in the body.

The kidneys and liver are two important organs that process and remove most drugs from the body. As we age, these organs may not work as well as they used to and drugs may leave more slowly.

Keep in mind that "drugs" can mean both medicines prescribed by your doctor and over-the-counter (OTC) medicines, which you buy without a doctor's prescription. OTCs can include vitamins and minerals, herbal and dietary supplements, laxatives, cold medicines, and antacids. Taking some OTCs together with prescription medicines can cause serious problems. For example, aspirin should not be taken with warfarin (Coumadin). Be sure your doctor knows what medicines you are taking and assures you that it is safe for you to take your medicines together. Also ask about taking your medicines with food. If you take alendronate (Fosamax) with food, for example, the drug will be less effective. Herbal supplements also should be taken with care. Gingko biloba, for instance, should not be taken with aspirin, acetaminophen, warfarin, or thiazide diuretics because it may increase blood pressure and the risk of bleeding problems.

You and your family should learn about the medicines that you take and their possible side effects. Remember, medicines that are strong enough to cure you can also be strong enough to hurt you if they aren't used correctly. Here are some hints to help avoid risks and get the best results from your medicines:

At Home

- DO keep a daily checklist of all the medicines you take. Include both prescription and OTC medicines. Note the name of each medicine, the doctor who prescribed it, the amount you take, and the times of day you take it. Keep a copy in your medicine cabinet and one in your wallet or pocketbook.

- DO read and save any written information that comes with the medicine.

- DO check the label on your medicine before taking it to make sure that it is for the correct person—you—with the correct directions prescribed for you by your doctor.

- DO take medicine in the exact amount and precise schedule your doctor prescribes.

- DO check the expiration dates on your medicine bottles and throw away medicine that has expired.

- DO call your doctor right away if you have any problems with your medicines or if you are worried that the medicine might be doing more harm than good. He or she may be able to change your medicine to another one that will work just as well.

- DO NOT take medicines prescribed for another person or give yours to someone else.

- DO NOT stop taking a prescription drug unless your doctor says it's okay—even if you are feeling better.

- DO NOT take more or less than the prescribed amount of any medicine.

- DO NOT mix alcohol and medicine unless your doctor says it's okay. Some medicines may not work well or may make you sick if taken with alcohol.

At Your Doctor's Office

- DO review your medicine record with the doctor or nurse at every visit and whenever your doctor prescribes new medicine. Your doctor may have new information about your medicines that might be important to you.

- DO always tell your doctor or nurse about past problems you have had with medicines, such as rashes, indigestion, dizziness, or not feeling hungry.

- DO always ask your doctor or nurse about the right way to take any medicine before you start to use it.

- DO ask these questions (and write down the answers) before leaving your doctor's office:

  ➤ What is the name of the medicine, and why am I taking it?

  ➤ What is the name of the condition this medicine will treat?

  ➤ How does this medicine work?

  ➤ How often should I take it?

  ➤ How long will it take to work?

  ➤ How will I know if this medicine is working?

  ➤ How can I expect to feel once I start taking this medicine?

  ➤ When should I take it? As needed? Before, with, or between meals? At bedtime?

  ➤ If I forget to take it, what should I do?

  ➤ What side effects might I expect? Should I report them?

  ➤ How long will I have to take it?

➤ Can this medicine interact with other medicines (prescription and OTCs including herbal and dietary supplements) that I am taking now?

➤ If I don't take medicine, is there anything else that would work as well?

At the Pharmacy

- DO make sure you can read and understand the medicine name and the directions on the container. If the label is hard to read, ask your pharmacist to use larger type. Let your pharmacist know if you have trouble opening the medicine bottle.

- DO check the label on your medicine before leaving the pharmacy to make sure that it is for the correct person—you—and with the correct directions prescribed for you by your doctor. If not, tell the pharmacist.

For More Information

The organizations listed below offer more information about some of the topics mentioned in this fact sheet:

The Food and Drug Administration (FDA), Consumer Affairs Office has more information about safe use of medicines.

Food and Drug Administration (FDA)
5600 Fishers Lane
HFD-210
Rockville, MD 20857
888-463-6332 (toll-free)
www.fda.gov

The Peter Lamy Center for Drug Therapy and Aging has brochures and information about medication use in the elderly. Contact:

University of Maryland School of Pharmacy
20 North Pine Street
Baltimore, MD 21201
410-706-7650

For more information about health and aging, contact:

National Institute on Aging Information Center
P.O. Box 8057
Gaithersburg, MD 20898-8057
800-222-2225 (toll-free)
800-222-4225 (TTY/toll-free)

- To order publications (in English or Spanish) online, visit www.niapublications.org.

- The National Institute on Aging website is www.nia.nih.gov.

- Visit NIHSeniorHealth.gov (www.nihseniorhealth.gov), a senior-friendly website from the National Institute on Aging and the National Library of Medicine. This simple-to-use website features popular health topics for older adults. It has large type and a "talking" function that reads the text out loud.

August 2000

Online Health Information: Can You Trust It?

A group of older adults are gathered for their weekly computer class. They are learning to use the Internet to find health information. Maria's husband, who is 75, had a stroke the month before so she's searching the Web for some basic facts about stroke rehabilitation. Walter, who is 68, has questions about what causes Alzheimer's disease because he thinks that's what his mother had. Shirley and Howard, married for 48 years, are trying to find out if the cataract surgery their eye doctor suggests really is as safe as he says. The whole group had one big worry—"How can we trust the health information we get on the Internet?"

There are thousands of health-related websites on the Internet. Some of the information on these websites is reliable and can be trusted. Some of it is not. Some of the information is current. Some of it is not. Choosing which website to trust is worth thinking about.

How Do I Find Reliable Health Information Online?

As a rule, health websites sponsored by Federal Government agencies are good sources of health information. You can reach all Federal websites by visiting *www.firstgov.gov*. Large professional organizations and well-known medical schools may also be good sources of health information.

The main page of a website is called the home page. The home page shows you the features on the website. You should be able to spot the name of the sponsor of the website right away.

Places to Start

There are a few good places to start if you are looking for online health information. An excellent source of reliable information is the National Institutes of Health (*www.nih.gov*). You can start here to find information on almost every health topic, including:

- Managing heart disease (*www.nhlbi.nih.gov*)
- Dealing with deafness (*www.nidcd.nih.gov*)
- Taking care of dentures (*www.nidcr.nih.gov*)
- Caring for a loved one with Alzheimer's disease (*www.nia.nih.gov*).

In addition, you can visit the National Library of Medicine's Medline Plus (*www.medlineplus.gov*) for dependable information on over 600 health-related topics.

You can also visit NIHSeniorHealth.gov (*www.nihseniorhealth.gov*)—a website with health information designed specifically for older people.

What Questions Should I Ask?

As you search online, you are likely to find websites for many health agencies and organizations that are not well-known. By answering the following questions you should be able to find more information about these websites. A lot of these details may be found under the heading, "About Us" or "Contact Us".

1. *Who sponsors the website? Can you easily identify the sponsor?*

Websites cost money—is the funding source readily apparent? Sometimes the website address itself may help— for example:

- .gov identifies a government agency,
- .edu identifies an educational institution,
- .org identifies professional organizations (e.g., scientific or research societies, advocacy groups), and
- .com identifies commercial websites (e.g., businesses, pharmaceutical companies, sometimes hospitals).

2. *Is it obvious how you can reach the sponsor?*

Trustworthy websites will have contact information for you to use. They often have a toll-free telephone number. The website home page should list an e-mail address, phone number, or a mailing address where the sponsor and/or the authors of the information can be reached.

3. *Who wrote the information?*

Authors and contributors should be identified. Their affiliation and any financial interest in the content should also be clear. Be careful about testimonials. Personal stories may be helpful, but medical advice offered in a case history should be considered with a healthy dose of skepticism. There is a big difference between a website developed by a person with a financial interest in a topic versus a website developed using strong scientific evidence. Reliable health information comes from scientific research that has been conducted in government, university, or private laboratories.

4. *Who reviews the information? Does the website have an editorial board?*

Click on the "About Us" page to see if there is an editorial board that checks the information before putting it online. Find out if the editorial board members are experts in the subject you are researching. For example, an advisory board made up of attorneys and accountants is not medically authoritative. Some websites have a section called, "About Our Writers" instead of an editorial policy. Dependable websites will tell you where the health information came from and how it has been reviewed.

5. *When was the information written?*

New research findings can make a difference in making medically smart choices. So, it's important to find out when the information you are reading was written. Look carefully on the home page to find out when the website was last updated. The date is often found at the bottom of the home page. Remember: older information isn't useless. Many websites provide older articles so readers can get an historical view of the information.

6. *Is your privacy protected? Does the website clearly state a privacy policy?*

This is important because, sadly, there is fraud on the Internet. Take time to read the website's policy—if the website says something like, "We share information with companies that can provide you with products," that's a sign your information isn't private. Do not give out your Social Security number. If you are asked for personal information, be sure to find out how the information is being used by contacting the website sponsor by phone, mail, or the "Contact Us" feature on the website. Be careful when buying things on the Internet. Websites without security may not protect your credit card or bank account information. Look for information saying that a website has a "secure server" before purchasing anything online.

7. *Does the website make claims that seem too good to be true? Are quick, miraculous cures promised?*

Be careful of claims that any one remedy will cure a lot of different illnesses. Be skeptical of sensational writing or dramatic cures.

Make sure you can find other websites with the same information. Don't be fooled by a long list of links—any website can link to another, so no endorsement can be implied from a shared link.

A Quick Checklist

You can use the following checklist to help make sure that the health information you are reading online can be trusted. You might want to keep this checklist by your computer.

1. Can you easily see who sponsors the website?

2. Is the sponsor a Federal agency or a medical school, or is it related to one of these?

3. Can you find the mission or goal of the sponsor of the website?

4. Can you see who works for the agency or organization and who is the author? Is there contact information?

5. Can you tell when the information was written?

6. Is your privacy protected?

7. Does the website make claims that seem too good to be true? Are quick, miraculous cures promised?

Take the "too good to be true" test—information that sounds unbelievable probably is unbelievable.

A Final Note

Use your common sense and good judgment when evaluating health information online. There are websites on nearly every conceivable health topic and no rules overseeing the quality of the information. Take a deep breath and think a bit before acting on any health information you find on the Web. Don't count on any one website. If possible, check with several sources to confirm the accuracy of your results. And remember to talk with your doctor.

For More Information

There are other resources that can help you identify good health information on the Internet. For more details, visit:

10 Questions to Help You Make Sense of Health Headlines
www.health-insight.com

Council of Better Business Bureaus
www.bbb.org

Health Internet Ethics
www.hiethics.org

Internet Health Coalition
www.ihealthcoalition.org

Medical Library Association
www.mlanet.org

National Library of Medicine MedlinePlus
www.medlineplus.gov

- In Health Topics, go to: "Evaluating Health Information"

QuackWatch
www.quackwatch.org

For more information about health and aging, contact:

National Institute on Aging Information Center
P.O. Box 8057
Gaithersburg, MD 20898-8057
800-222-2225 (toll-free)
800-222-4225 (TTY/toll-free)

- To order publications (in English or Spanish) online, visit www.niapublications.org.
- The National Institute on Aging website is www.nia.nih.gov.
- Visit NIHSeniorHealth.gov (www.nihseniorhealth.gov), a senior-friendly website from the National Institute on Aging and the National Library of Medicine. This simple-to-use website features popular health topics for older adults. It has large type and a "talking" function that reads the text out loud.

2003

Staying Safe and Planning Ahead

How to protect yourself now and plan for the future

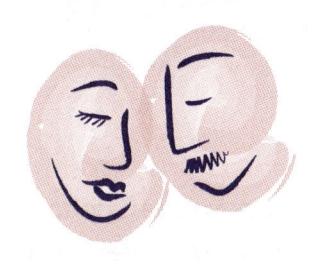

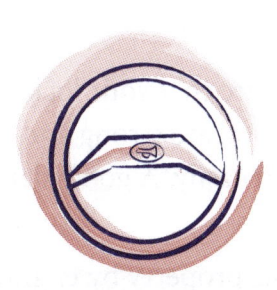

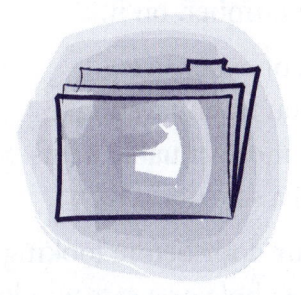

158 **Crime and Older People**

162 **Getting Your Affairs in Order**

166 **Hyperthermia—Too Hot for Your Health**

170 **Hypothermia: A Cold Weather Hazard**

175 **Long-Term Care: Choosing the Right Place**

180 **Older Drivers**

184 **Preventing Falls and Fractures**

Crime and Older People

> Lucy is worried. She's lived in the old neighborhood for 50 years, but things seem to be changing. Last week her friend Rose was walking to the store when a young man ran by and pulled her purse right off her shoulder. Two weeks ago Joe, the man upstairs, said he put his grocery bags on the curb while waiting for the bus, and before he knew it, someone had picked up his bags and run off.
>
> Lucy feels sad to think she might have to move. She wonders, is anywhere safe for older people anymore?

Older people and their families worry about crime. Though older people are less likely to be victims of crime than teenagers and young adults, the number of crimes against older people is hard to ignore. It is often highly publicized. Each year, over two million older people are victims of crime.

Older people are often targets for robbery, purse snatching, pocket picking, car theft, or home repair scams. They are more likely than younger people to face attackers who are strangers. During a crime, an older person is more likely to be seriously hurt than someone who is younger.

But, even though there are risks, don't let a fear of crime stop you from enjoying life. Be careful, and be aware of your surroundings. The following is a general overview of some of the areas of most concern to older people. These are common sense tips that can help fight crime and protect your safety. At the end of the fact sheet you can find a list of resources that will have a lot more information that can help.

Stay Safe

There are a lot of things you can do to keep you, your money, and your property safe. These do's and don'ts give you a place to start:

Be safe at home

- Do try to make sure that your locks, doors, and windows are strong and cannot be broken easily. A good alarm system can help.

- Do mark valuable property by engraving an identification number, such as your driver's license number, on it.

- Do make a list of expensive belongings—you might even take pictures of the most valuable items. Store these details in a safe place.

- Don't open your door before looking through the peephole or a safe window to see who's there. Ask any stranger to show proof that he or she is who they claim to be. Remember, you don't have to open the door if you feel uneasy.

- Don't keep large amounts of money in the house.
- Do get to know your neighbors—join a Neighborhood Watch Program.

Be street smart

- Do try to stay alert. Walk with a friend. Stay away from unsafe places like dark parking lots or alleys. If you drive, don't open your door or roll down your window for strangers. Park in well-lit areas.
- Do have your monthly pension or Social Security checks sent right to the bank for direct deposit. Try not to have a regular banking routine.
- Don't carry a lot of cash. Put your wallet, money, or credit cards in an inside pocket. Carry your purse close to your body with the strap over your shoulder and across your chest.
- Do not resist a robber—hand over your cash right away.
- Don't keep your check book and credit cards together. A thief who steals both could use the card to forge your signature on checks.

Fight Fraud

Older people may be victims of fraud, such as con games, insurance scams, home repair scams, and/or telephone and Internet scams. Even trusted friends or family members can steal an older person's money or property. Trust what you feel. The following tips may help:

Be smart with your money

- Don't be afraid to hang up the phone on telephone salespeople. Remember, you can always say no to any offer. You aren't being impolite—you are taking care of yourself!
- Don't give any personal information, including your credit card number or bank account, over the phone unless you have made the phone call. Be careful when returning a sales call.
- Don't take money from your bank account if a stranger tells you to. In one common swindle a thief pretends to be a bank employee and asks you to take out money to "test" a bank teller. Banks do not check their employees this way.
- Don't be fooled by deals that "are too good to be true." They are often scams. Beware of deals that ask for a lot of money up front and promise you success. Check with your local Better Business Bureau to get more information about the reliability of a company.
- Do be on guard about hiring people that come door-to-door looking for home repair work. They may overcharge you. You should try to check their references. Always spell out the details of the work you want done in writing. Never pay for the whole job in advance.

Avoid Identity Theft

How can someone steal your identity? If they use your name, Social Security number, or credit card without your go-ahead—that's called identity theft, and it's a serious crime.

Protect yourself

- Do take care to keep information about your checking account private—keep all new and cancelled checks in a safe place; report any stolen checks right away; carefully look at your monthly bank account statement.

- Do shred everything that has personal information about you written on it.

- Do be very careful when buying things online. Websites without security may not protect your credit card or bank account information. Look for information saying that a website has a 'secure server' before buying anything online.

Elder Abuse—It's a Crime

It's hard to believe, but elder abuse can happen anywhere—at home by family or friends or in a nursing home by professional caregivers. Many people don't think of elder abuse as a crime, but it is. In addition to physical harm, abuse can include taking financial advantage, neglecting, sexually abusing, or abandoning an older person. Most abuse involves verbal threats or hurtful words. It only rarely involves weapons or causes physical injury beyond minor cuts and bruises. If someone you know is being abused, or if you need help, remember:

- You can help yourself and others by reporting the crimes when they happen. If you do not report a crime because of embarrassment or fear the criminal stays on the streets. Reporting abuse is a moral as well as legal responsibility in most states.

- Contact your local or state Adult Protective Service programs for help.

- If you have been hurt, go to a doctor as soon as possible. Even though you may not see anything wrong, there is always the possibility of internal damage.

- Contact a lawyer. He or she will assist you in any legal action that needs to be taken.

- Plan for your own future. Arrange a health-related power of attorney (also called an advance directive) or have a living will so your family knows your wishes for the future.

For More Information

There are many organizations that have more in-depth information on crime prevention or protection. Check with the following groups for suggestions that can help you feel safer:

National Organization for Victim Assistance
510 King Street, Suite 424
Alexandria, VA 23314
800-879-6682 (toll-free)
www.trynova.org

- 24-hour hotline

AARP-Consumer Protection
601 E Street, NW
Washington, DC 20049
202-434-2222
www.aarp.org/consumerprotect

US Council of Better Business Bureaus
4200 Wilson Boulevard
Suite 800
Arlington, VA 22203-1838
www.bbb.org

Federal Trade Commission
600 Pennsylvania Avenue, NW
Washington, DC 20580
877-382-4387 (toll-free)
www.ftc.gov

- Look for the booklet *When Bad Things Happen to Your Good Name*

National Domestic Violence Hotline
800-799-7233 (toll-free)
800-787-3224 (TTD/toll-free)

- 24 hours/day, 365 days/year

National Center on Elder Abuse
1201 15th Street, NW, Suite 350
Washington, DC 20005-2800
202-898-2586
www.elderabusecenter.org

For more information about health and aging, contact:

National Institute on Aging Information Center
P.O. Box 8057
Gaithersburg, MD 20898-8057
800-222-2225 (toll-free)
800-222-4225 (TTY/toll-free)

- To order publications (in English or Spanish) online, visit *www.niapublications.org*.
- The National Institute on Aging website is *www.nia.nih.gov*.
- Visit NIHSeniorHealth.gov (*www.nihseniorhealth.gov*), a senior-friendly website from the National Institute on Aging and the National Library of Medicine. This simple-to-use website features popular health topics for older adults. It has large type and a "talking" function that reads the text out loud.

2003

Getting Your Affairs in Order

Ben has been married for 50 years. He always managed the family's money. But since his stroke Ben can't walk or talk. Shirley, his wife, feels overwhelmed. Of course, she's worried about Ben's health. But, on top of that, she has no idea what bills should be paid or when they are due.

Eighty-year-old Louise lives alone. One night she fell in the kitchen and broke her hip. She spent one week in the hospital and two months in an assisted living facility. Even though her son lives across the country, he was able to pay her bills and handle her Medicare questions right away. That's because several years ago, Louise and her son talked about what to do in case of a medical emergency.

Plan for the Future

No one ever plans to be sick or disabled. Yet it's just this kind of planning that can make all the difference in an emergency. Long before she fell, Louise had put all her important papers in one place and told her son where to find them. She gave him the name of her lawyer as well as a list of people he could contact at her bank, doctor's office, investment firm, and insurance company. She made sure he had copies of her Medicare and other health insurance cards. She added her son's name to her checking account, allowing him to write checks on her account. Finally, Louise made sure Medicare and her doctor had written permission to talk with her son about her health or any insurance claims.

On the other hand, because Ben always took care of family financial matters, he never talked about the details with Shirley. No one but Ben knew that his life insurance policy was in a box in the closet or that the car title and deed to the house were filed in his desk drawer. Ben never expected his wife would have to take over. His lack of planning has made a tough situation even tougher for Shirley.

Steps for Getting Your Affairs in Order

- Gather everything you can about your income, investments, insurance, and savings.
- Put your important papers and copies of legal documents in one place. You could set up a file, put everything in a desk or dresser drawer, or just list the information and location of papers in a notebook. If your papers are in a bank safe deposit box, keep copies in a file at home. Check each year to see if there's anything new to add.
- Tell a trusted family member or friend where you put all your important papers. You don't need to tell this friend or family member your personal business,

but someone should know where you keep your papers in case of emergency. If you don't have a relative or friend you trust, ask a lawyer to help.

- Give consent in advance for your doctor or lawyer to talk with your caregiver as needed. There may be questions about your care, a bill, or a health insurance claim. Without your consent, your caregiver may not be able to get needed information. You can give permission in advance to Medicare, a credit card company, your bank, or your doctor. Sometimes you can give your OK over the telephone. Other times you may need to sign and return a form.

Legal Documents

There are many different types of legal documents that can help you plan how your affairs will be handled in the future:

- *Wills* and *trusts* give you a way to say how you want the things you own given out after you die.

- *Advance directives* describe your health care wishes in case you can't speak for yourself. Advance directives such as a *living will* or *durable power of attorney for health care* can say how you want your health managed and may help avoid family conflict over your care. They also may make it easier for family members to make hard health care decisions on your behalf. For example, your aunt may not wish to have her life extended by being placed on a breathing machine (ventilator), or your brother may want to be an organ donor. Advance directives help people plan for these situations. Different states have different forms for advance directives.

- A *power of attorney* lets you give someone the authority to act on your behalf. There are different types:
  - A *standard power of attorney* lets you name another person to handle your

Personal Records

- **Full legal name**
- **Social Security number**
- **Legal residence**
- **Date and place of birth**
- **Names and addresses of spouse and children (or location of death certificates)**
- **Location of "living will" or other advance directive**
- **Location of birth certificate and certificates of marriage, divorce, citizenship, and adoption**
- **Employers and dates of employment**
- **Medications you take regularly**
- **Education and military records**
- **Your religion, name of church or synagogue, and names of clergy**
- **Memberships in groups and awards received**
- **Names and addresses of close friends, relatives, doctors, clergy, and lawyers or financial advisor**

personal or financial matters. This is useful only if you can still make your own decisions.

- A *durable power of attorney* lets you name another person to make decisions for you if you become unable to make your own decisions.

- A *durable power of attorney for health care* lets you name another person to make medical decisions for you if you are unable to make them yourself.

■ A *living will* says how you want your health care handled if you are in a life threatening situation and cannot make medical decisions for yourself. It gives you the right to refuse certain types of care. It also gives those caring for you the legal right to follow your wishes.

State laws vary, so check with your area office on aging, a lawyer, or a financial planner about the rules and requirements in your state.

What Exactly is an *"Important Paper"*?

The answer to this question may be different for every family. The lists here can help you decide what is important for you. Remember, this is just a starting point. You may have other information to add. For example, if you have a pet, be sure to

Financial Records

- **Sources of income and assets (pension funds, IRAs, 401Ks, interest, etc.)**
- **Information about insurance policies, bank accounts, deeds, investments, and other valuables, such as jewelry or art**
- **Social Security and Medicare information**
- **Investment income (stocks, bonds, property) and stockbrokers' names and addresses**
- **Insurance information (life, health, long-term care, home, and car) with policy numbers and agents' names**
- **Name of your bank and bank account numbers (checking, savings, and credit union)**
- **Location of safe deposit boxes**
- **Copy of most recent income tax return**
- **Copy of your will**
- **Liabilities—what you owe, to whom, and when payments are due**
- **Mortgages and debts—how and when paid**
- **Location of deed of trust and car title**
- **Credit card and charge account names and numbers**
- **Property tax information**
- **Location of all personal items, such as jewelry and family treasures**

BOUND FOR YOUR GOOD HEALTH: A COLLECTION OF AGE PAGES

include the name and address of your vet or someone who could care for him or her.

If Your Caregiver Lives Far Away

The person you choose to help you may live far away. In that case, a little more information can make it easier for him or her to help. For example, make sure she or he has the names, phone numbers, and e-mail addresses of people near you who could be helpful in an emergency, such as:

- Family members, friends, and neighbors who live nearby,
- Your apartment manager,
- Your doctor and other health care providers,
- Your clergy, or
- Your lawyer, accountant, or other advisors.

Update this information every year.

Resources

You may want to talk with a lawyer about setting up a power of attorney, durable power of attorney, joint account, trust, or advance directive. Be sure to ask about the cost before you make an appointment. You should be able to find a directory of local lawyers at your library. An informed family member may be able to help you manage some of these issues.

For More Information

The following organizations may be helpful:

AARP
601 E Street, NW
Washington, DC 20049
800-304-4222 (toll-free)
www.aarp.org

National Association of Area Agencies on Aging
1730 Rhode Island Avenue, NW
Washington, DC 20036
202-842-0888
www.n4a.org

National Association of State Units on Aging
1201 15th Street, NW, Suite 350
Washington, DC 20005
202-898-2578
www.nasua.org

Centers for Medicare and Medicaid Services
7500 Security Boulevard
Baltimore, MD 21244-1850
877-267-2323 (toll-free)
866-226-1819 (TTY/toll-free)
www.cms.gov

For more information about health and aging, contact:

National Institute on Aging Information Center
P.O. Box 8057
Gaithersburg, MD 20898-8057
800-222-2225 (toll-free)
800-222-4225 (TTY/toll-free)

- To order publications (in English or Spanish) online, visit www.niapublications.org.

- The National Institute on Aging website is www.nia.nih.gov.
- Visit NIHSeniorHealth.gov (www.nihseniorhealth.gov), a senior-friendly website from the National Institute on Aging and the National Library of Medicine. This simple-to-use website features popular health topics for older adults. It has large type and a "talking" function that reads the text out loud.

June 2004

GETTING YOUR AFFAIRS IN ORDER 165

Hyperthermia—Too Hot for Your Health

Irene used to be a schoolteacher. Now retired, she loves to work in her garden. Because she has always spent hours outside, digging, weeding, and planting, she believes the heat and humidity of midwestern summers doesn't bother her. Then last year an unusual heat wave hit her area for a week. Every day the temperature was over 100°F, and the humidity was at least 90 percent. Irene's house only has one large fan. It just wasn't enough to fight the effect of the heat and humidity on her body. Five days into the heat wave, her daughter came over because Irene sounded confused on the phone. She found her mom passed out on the kitchen floor. The ambulance came quickly when called, but Irene almost died. She had heat stroke, the most serious form of hyperthermia.

Almost every summer there is a deadly heat wave in some part of the country. Too much heat is not safe for anyone. It is even riskier if you are older or if you have health problems. It is important to get relief from the heat quickly. If not, you might begin to feel confused or faint. Your heart could become stressed, and sometimes this causes death.

Your body is always working to keep a balance between how much heat it makes and how much it loses. Your brain is the thermostat. It sends and receives signals to and from parts of your body that affect temperature, such as the spinal cord, muscles, blood vessels, skin, and glands that make substances known as hormones. Too much heat causes sweating. When the sweat dries from your skin, the surface of your body cools, and your temperature goes down.

Being in heat for too long can cause many illnesses, all grouped under the name *hyperthermia* (hy-per-ther-mee-uh):

- *Heat cramps* are the painful tightening of muscles in your stomach area, arms, or legs. Cramps can result from hard work or exercise. While your body temperature and pulse usually stay normal during heat cramps, your skin may feel moist and cool. Take these cramps as a sign that you are too hot—find a way to cool your body down. Be sure to drink plenty of fluids, but not those containing alcohol or caffeine.

- *Heat edema* is a swelling in your ankles and feet when you get hot. Putting your legs up should help. If that doesn't work fairly quickly, check with your doctor.

- *Heat syncope* is a sudden dizziness that may come on when you are active in the heat.

If you take a form of heart medication known as a beta blocker or are not used to hot weather, you are even more likely to feel faint when in the heat. Putting your legs up and resting in a cool place should make the dizzy feeling go away.

- *Heat exhaustion* is a warning that your body can no longer keep itself cool in the hot air surrounding it. You might feel thirsty, dizzy, weak, uncoordinated, nauseated, and sweat a lot. Your body temperature is still normal, and your pulse might be normal or raised. Your skin feels cold and clammy. Resting in a cool place, drinking plenty of fluids, and getting medical care should help you feel better soon. If not, this condition can progress to heat stroke.

- *Heat stroke* is an emergency—it can be **life threatening**! You need to get medical help right away. Getting to a cool place is very important, but so is treatment by a doctor. Many people die of heat stroke each year. Older people living in homes or apartments without air conditioning or good airflow are at most risk. So are people who don't drink enough water or those with chronic diseases or alcoholism.

Who Is at Risk?

Around 200 people die each year during very hot weather. Most are over 50 years old. The temperature outside or inside does not have to hit 100°F for you to be at risk for a heat-related illness. Health problems that put you at risk include:

- Heart or blood vessel problems, poorly working sweat glands, or changes in your skin caused by normal aging,

The Signs of Heat Stroke

- **Fainting, possibly the first sign,**
- **Body temperature over 104° F,**
- **A change in behavior—confusion, being grouchy, acting strangely, or staggering,**
- **Dry flushed skin and a strong rapid pulse or a slow weak pulse, and**
- **Not sweating, despite the heat, acting delirious, or being in a coma.**

- Heart, lung, or kidney disease, as well as any illness that makes you feel weak all over or causes a fever,

- High blood pressure or other conditions that make it necessary for you to change some of the foods you eat. For example, if you are supposed to avoid salt in your food, your risk of heat-related illness may be higher. Check with your doctor.

- Conditions treated by drugs such as diuretics, sedatives, tranquilizers, and some heart and blood pressure medicines. These may make it harder for your body to cool itself by perspiring.

- Taking several drugs for a variety of health problems. Keep taking your prescriptions, but ask your doctor what to do if the drugs you are taking make you more likely to become overheated.

- Being quite a bit overweight or underweight, or

- Drinking alcoholic beverages.

How Can I Lower My Risk?

Things you can do to lower your risk of heat-related illness:

- Drink plenty of liquids—water or fruit and vegetable juices. Every day you should drink at least eight glasses to keep your body working properly. Heat tends to make you lose fluids so it is very important to drink at least that much, if not more, when it is hot. Avoid drinks containing caffeine or alcohol. They make you lose more fluids. If your doctor has told you to limit your liquids, ask him or her what you should do when it is very hot.

- If you live in a home or apartment without fans or air conditioning, be sure to follow these steps to lower your chance of heat problems:
  - Open windows at night,
  - Create cross-ventilation by opening windows on two sides of the building,
  - Cover windows when they are in direct sunlight, and
  - Keep curtains, shades, or blinds drawn during the hottest part of the day.

- Try to spend at least two hours a day (if possible during the hottest part of the day) some place air-conditioned—for example, the shopping mall, the movies, the library, a senior center, or a friend's house if you don't have air conditioning.

- Check with your local Area Agency on Aging to see if there is a program that provides window air conditioners to seniors who qualify.

- If you think you can't afford to run your air conditioner in the summer, contact your local Area Agency on Aging. Or, ask at your local senior center. They may know if there are any programs in your community to aid people who need help paying their cooling bills. The Low Income Home Energy Assistance Program (LIHEAP) is one possible source.

- Ask a friend or relative to drive you to a cool place on very hot days if you don't have a car or no longer drive. Many towns or counties, area agencies, religious groups, and senior citizen centers provide such services. If necessary, take a taxi. **Don't** stand outside waiting for a bus.

- Pay attention to the weather reports. You are more at risk as the temperature or humidity rise or when there is an air pollution alert in effect.

- Dress for the weather. Some people find natural fabrics such as cotton to be cooler than synthetic fibers. Light-colored clothes reflect the sun and heat better than dark colors. If you are unsure about what to wear, ask a friend or family member to help you select clothing that will help you stay cool.

- **Don't** try to exercise or do a lot of activities when it is hot.

- Avoid crowded places when it's hot outside. Plan trips during non-rush hour times.

What Should I Remember?

Headache, confusion, dizziness, or nausea when you're in a hot place or during hot weather—these could be a sign of a heat-related illness. Go to the doctor or an emergency room to find out if these are caused by the heat or not. To keep heat-related illnesses from becoming dangerous heat stroke, remember to:

- Get out of the sun and into a cool place—it would be best if it is air-conditioned.
- Offer fluids, but avoid alcohol and caffeine. Water and fruit and vegetable juices are best.
- Shower or bathe, or at least sponge off with cool water.
- Lie down and rest, if possible in a cool place.
- Visit your doctor or an emergency room if you don't cool down quickly.

For More Information

These organizations offer information about hyperthermia and related services:

Eldercare Locator:
800-677-1116 (toll-free)
www.eldercare.gov

Low Income Home Energy Assistance Program (LIHEAP)
National Energy Assistance Referral Hotline (NEAR)
866-674-6327 (toll-free)
www.ncat.org

To find your local Area Agency on Aging look in the telephone book or contact:
National Association of Area Agencies on Aging
1730 Rhode Island Avenue, NW
Suite 1200
Washington, DC 20036
202-872-0888
www.n4a.org

For more information about health and aging, contact:
National Institute on Aging Information Center
P.O. Box 8057
Gaithersburg, MD 20898-8057
800-222-2225 (toll-free)
800-222-4225 (TTY/toll-free)

- To order publications (in English or Spanish) online, visit *www.niapublications.org*.
- The National Institute on Aging website is *www.nia.nih.gov*.
- Visit NIHSeniorHealth.gov (*www.nihseniorhealth.gov*), a senior-friendly website from the National Institute on Aging and the National Library of Medicine. This simple-to-use website features popular health topics for older adults. It has large type and a "talking" function that reads the text out loud.

July 2001

Hypothermia: A Cold Weather Hazard

Tony is a retired mailman. He has lived in New England his whole life and has seen some harsh winters. None, however, was as cold or snowy as one winter a few years ago. First, the temperature dipped to below zero and a snowstorm left two feet of snow. Then an ice storm caused lots of broken power lines. That meant Tony had no heat in his house, but he also couldn't leave. The temperature inside dropped to 60°F quite quickly. When his neighbor rang the doorbell to check on him the next day, Tony was confused, and his speech was slurred. He was taken to the emergency room. A doctor examined him and warmed him up. Tony went to his brother's house until the heat came back on. Turns out he'd had accidental hypothermia.

Cold weather is very risky for older people. Almost everyone knows about winter dangers such as broken bones from falls on ice or breathing problems caused by cold air. But the winter chill can also lower the temperature inside your body. That can be deadly if not treated quickly. This drop in body temperature, often caused by staying in a cool place for too long, is called *hypothermia* (hi-po-ther-mee-uh).

A body temperature below 96°F may seem like just a couple of degrees below the body's normal temperature of 98.6°F. It can be dangerous. It may cause an irregular heartbeat leading to heart problems and death.

What to Look For

When you think about being cold, you probably think of shivering. That is one thing the body does when it gets cold. This warms the body. Muscles shiver in response to messages sent by the nerves. Shivering increases muscle cell activity that, in turn, makes heat. But, shivering alone does not mean hypothermia.

So, how can you tell if someone has hypothermia? It can be tricky because some older people may not want to complain. They may not even be aware of how cold it is. Look for the "*umbles*"—*stumbles*, *mumbles*, *fumbles*, and *grumbles*—these show that the cold is affecting how well a person's muscles and nerves work. Watch for:

- Confusion or sleepiness,
- Slowed, slurred speech or shallow breathing,
- Weak pulse or low blood pressure,
- A change in behavior during cold weather or a change in the way they look,

- A lot of shivering or no shivering; stiffness in the arms or legs,
- Chilly rooms or other signs that they have been in a cold place, or
- Poor control over body movements or slow reactions.

What Should I Do?

If you think someone could have hypothermia, take his or her temperature with a thermometer. Make sure you shake the thermometer so it starts below its lowest point. If the temperature doesn't rise above 96°F, call for emergency help. In many areas that means calling 911.

The only way to tell for sure that someone has hypothermia is to use a special thermometer that can read very low body temperatures. Most hospitals have such thermometers. The person **must** be seen by a doctor. If possible, the doctor should know about hypothermia and work in a well-equipped hospital emergency room. There, the doctors will warm the person's body from inside out. For example, they may give the person warm fluids directly into a vein using an I.V. Whether the person gets better depends on how long he or she was exposed to the cold and his or her general health.

While you are waiting for help to arrive, keep the person warm and dry. Move him or her to a warmer place, if possible. Wrap the person in blankets, towels, coats—whatever is handy. Even your own body warmth will help. Lie close, but be gentle. You may be tempted to rub the person's arms and legs. This can make the problem worse. The skin of an older person may be thinner and more easily torn than the skin of someone younger.

What Things Put Me at Risk?

Some things that put any older person at risk for hypothermia and some things you can do to avoid it include:

- Changes in your body that come with aging can make it harder to feel when you are getting cold. It may be harder for your body to warm itself. Pay attention to how cold it is where you are.
- If you don't eat well, you might have less fat under your skin. Fat can protect your body. It keeps heat in your body. Make sure you are eating enough food to keep up your weight.
- Some illnesses may make it harder for your body to stay warm. These include:
  - Disorders of the body's hormone system such as low thyroid (hypothyroidism),
  - Any condition that interferes with the normal flow of blood such as diabetes, and
  - Some skin problems such as psoriasis that allow your body to lose more heat than normal. Regularly visit your doctor who can keep any illness

under control, and try to stay away from cold places.

- Other health problems might keep you from moving to a warmer place or putting on more clothes or a blanket. For example:
  ➤ Severe arthritis, Parkinson's disease, or other illnesses that make it harder to move around,
  ➤ Stroke or other illnesses that can leave you paralyzed and make clear thinking more difficult,
  ➤ Memory disorders or dementia, and
  ➤ A fall or other injury.

- Some medicines often used by older people also increase the risk of accidental hypothermia. These include drugs used to treat anxiety, depression, or nausea. Some over-the-counter cold remedies can also cause problems. Ask your doctor how the medicines you are taking affect body heat.

- Alcoholic drinks can also make you lose body heat faster. Use alcohol moderately, if at all. Do not drink alcohol before bedtime when it gets colder outside—and maybe inside, too.

- Clothing can make you colder or help keep you warm. Tight clothing can keep your blood from flowing freely. This can lead to loss of body heat. Wear several layers of loose clothing when it is cold. The layers will trap warm air between them.

Staying Warm Inside and Out

Maybe you already knew that your health, your age, what you eat or drink, even your clothes can make it hard for you to stay warm enough wherever you are. What you might not realize is that people can also get cold enough inside a building to get very sick. In fact, hypothermia can even happen to someone in a nursing home or group facility if the rooms are not kept warm enough. People living there who are already sick may have special problems keeping warm. If someone you know is in a group facility, pay attention to the inside temperature there and to whether that person is dressed warmly enough.

Homes or apartments that are not heated enough, even with a temperature of 60°F to 65°F, can lead to illness. This is a special problem if you live alone because there is no one else to comment on the chilliness of the house or to notice if you are having symptoms of hypothermia. Set your thermostat for at least 68°F to 70°F. If a power outage leaves you without heat, try to stay with a relative or friend.

Avoid using space heaters if your home seems cold or if you want to keep the thermostat set lower to keep your heating costs down. Some types are fire hazards, and others can cause carbon monoxide poisoning. The U.S. Consumer Product Safety Commission has information on the use of space heaters, but here are a few things to remember:

- Make sure your space heater has been approved by a recognized testing laboratory.
- Choose the right size heater for the space you are heating.
- Keep substances that can catch fire like paint, pets, clothing, towels, curtains, and papers away from the heating element.
- Keep the door to the rest of the house open for good air flow.
- Turn the heater off when you leave the room or go to bed.
- Make sure your smoke alarms are working.
- Put a carbon monoxide detector near where people sleep.
- Keep the right type of fire extinguisher nearby.

Don't forget that you need to stay warm when it's cold outside. Remember that this means knowing if weather forecasts are for very cold temperatures or for windy and cold weather. You lose more body heat on a windy day than a calm day. Weather forecasters call this the wind-chill factor. They often suggest, even when the outside temperature itself is not very low, that the wind-chill factor is cold enough for people to stay indoors. If you must go out, dress correctly. Be sure to wear a hat and gloves, as well as warm clothes.

Is There Help for My Heating Bills?

Sometimes older people need help making sure their home will keep them warm enough. Some help is available. If your home doesn't have enough insulation, contact your state or local energy agency or the local power or gas company. They can give you information about weatherizing your home. This can help keep the heating bills down. You might also think about only heating the rooms you use in the house. For example, shut the heating vents and doors to any bedrooms not being used. Keep the door to the basement closed.

If you have a limited income, you may qualify for help paying your heating bill. State and local energy agencies or gas and electric companies may have special programs. Another possible source of help is the Low Income Home Energy Assistance Program (LIHEAP). This program supports some people with small incomes who need help paying their heating and cooling bills. Your local Area Agency on Aging, senior center, or community action agency may have information on programs such as these.

Are you worried that your landlord may want to cut off the gas or electricity in cold weather if you cannot pay a utility bill? Many states and cities now have laws to protect you, at least until other plans are made. Do not wait for winter to find out about these programs. Check with your local government about the laws that may apply where you live.

For More Information The organizations listed below offer more information about some of the topics mentioned in this fact sheet:

U.S. Consumer Product Safety Commission
Washington, DC 20207-0001
800-638-2772 (toll-free)
800-638-8270 (TTY/toll-free)
www.cpsc.gov

To find your local Area Agency on Aging look in the telephone book or contact:

National Association of Area Agencies on Aging
1730 Rhode Island Avenue, NW
Suite 1200
Washington, DC 20036
202-872-0888
www.n4a.org

Eldercare Locator
800-677-1116 (toll-free)
www.eldercare.gov

Low Income Home Energy Assistance Program (LIHEAP)
National Energy Assistance Referral Hotline (NEAR)
866-674-6327 (toll-free)
www.ncat.org

For more information about health and aging, contact:

National Institute on Aging Information Center
P.O. Box 8057
Gaithersburg, MD 20898-8057
800-222-2225 (toll-free)
800-222-4225 (TTY/toll-free)

- To order publications (in English or Spanish) online, visit www.niapublications.org.
- The National Institute on Aging website is www.nia.nih.gov.
- Visit NIHSeniorHealth.gov (www.nihseniorhealth.gov), a senior-friendly website from the National Institute on Aging and the National Library of Medicine. This simple-to-use website features popular health topics for older adults. It has large type and a "talking" function that reads the text out loud.

August 2001

Long-Term Care: Choosing the Right Place

Many of us hope to stay in our homes as we grow older. Often we are able to do that. But later in life—usually by our 80s and 90s—some of us need a hand with everyday activities like shopping, cooking, or bathing. A few of us need more help on a regular basis. Maybe that means it's time to move to a place where expert care is available around-the-clock.

Where to Start

Do you think that your family member can't live at home any longer? It might be your husband or wife, a parent, aunt or uncle, or even a grandparent. You've added a handrail on the front steps and grab bars in the bathroom. You made plans for a home health aide to come to the house every day. You arranged for help with meals, and you visit every day. But now you wonder if staying at home is the best choice. Where do you go for help? Here are some answers to that and other questions that you might have as you look for the best place for you or your relative to live.

Sometimes the need for help grows over time. For example, Bob is 87 years old. He has lived alone since his wife died ten years ago. For the last few years, he has needed more and more help doing things for himself. First, he had trouble making meals. So, he ate a big lunch at the local senior center until last year when he gave up driving. Now sometimes his daughter drops off meals. Other times meals are delivered by a local program. The stairs in his house are getting too hard to climb. Bob also forgets more and more things. He often forgets to take his blood pressure medicine. He has also left the burner on the stove turned on several times. He doesn't want to move in with his daughter and her family, so Bob and his daughter are looking for a new place for him to live.

Over the last year Bob's daughter has been thinking this time might come. She knows what's available. She's looked into how they will pay for the care her dad needs. Bob too has been doing some planning. He is sad about leaving his home, but he has been preparing for the time when he'd need more help. He even put his name on a waiting list for a nearby retirement community that he liked. Now they have an opening there. The admission coordinator at the community will help him decide if he can live in one of their apartments or needs to be in their assisted living facility.

Bob and his daughter were lucky. Sometimes you need to make a choice quickly. If you haven't planned ahead, then making a decision might not be so easy. For example, Alice and her husband have lived in their house for 50 years. At 84, she still loves to cook and work in her garden every day. Last week she slipped in her bathroom, fell, and broke her hip. Now after an operation to fix her hip, she needs to go somewhere for nursing care and rehabilitation. Her doctors don't know if she'll ever recover enough to go home again. Her children live hundreds of miles away. But her husband and family only have a few days to find a place.

Alice and her family were not prepared like Bob and his family. The social worker and discharge planner at the hospital will help them find a place for Alice to go for therapy after she leaves the hospital. But if she is too frail to go home after her hip heals, she and her family will have to choose a place for her to live permanently.

What Are the Choices?

There are two kinds of senior living facilities based on how much help is needed:

- Assisted living facilities, and
- Skilled nursing facilities or nursing homes.

You should think about an *assisted living facility* if you or your relative don't need a lot of medical care but do need more help than can easily be gotten at home. Assisted living homes can give someone as much help as needed with daily living, but offer only some nursing care or none at all. People often live independently in their own unit. The place provides meals and house cleaning, offers interesting things to do, and takes residents wherever they need to go, like the doctor or the shopping mall. They can also provide help with bathing, dressing, and taking medicines, if needed.

Some assisted living facilities are part of a *continuing care retirement community* or *lifecare community*. These communities offer independent living and skilled nursing facilities as well as assisted living. Sometimes assisted living help is set up in a home with only a few residents. These are often called *board and care homes*.

If your relative becomes very frail or suffers from the later stages of dementia, more care could be needed. A *nursing home* or *skilled nursing facility* may be necessary if someone:

- Needs round-the-clock nursing care,
- Might wander away without supervision,
- Needs help with meals, bathing, personal care, medications, and moving around,
- Needs more help than the current caregiver can possibly give, or
- Cannot live alone.

These places supply 24-hour services and supervision, including medical care and some physical, speech, and occupational therapy, to people living there. They might also offer other services such as social activities and transportation. As a rule, the rooms are for one or two people. Some places want residents to bring some special items from home to make their rooms more familiar. Some even allow a pet or make it possible for couples to stay together.

Both assisted living and skilled nursing facilities sometimes offer special areas for people with dementia. These areas are designed to meet the special needs of these people and to keep them safe from wandering.

How to Choose

Ask questions. Find out what is available in your area. Is there any place close enough for family and friends to visit easily? Doctors, friends and relatives, local hospital discharge planners and social workers, and religious organizations may know of places.

Also, each state has a *Long-Term Care Ombudsman*. They have information and may be able to answer questions about a place you are considering. The ombudsman is also available to help solve problems that might come up between a nursing home and the resident or the family. To find your state long-term care ombudsman, contact the Administration on Aging's *Eldercare Locator* at 800-677-1116 or www.eldercare.gov.

Is the person in need of long-term care a military veteran? They might be able to get help through the Department of Veterans Affairs programs. You can check by going to www.va.gov, calling the VA Health Care Benefits number, 877-222-8387, or contacting the VA medical center nearest you.

Call. Once you have a list of possible places, get in touch with each one. Ask basic questions about openings and waiting lists, number of residents, costs and methods of payment, and their link to Medicare and Medicaid. Take a few minutes to think about what's important to you or your relative, such as transportation, meals, activities, connection to a certain religion, or special units for Alzheimer's disease.

Visit. Make plans to meet with the director of nursing and director of social services. Medicare offers a nursing home checklist to use when visiting (see *Help in Planning*). Some of the things to look for include certification for Medicare and Medicaid, handicap access, no strong odors (either bad or good ones), contact between staff and current residents, volunteers, and the appearance of residents. If the nursing home is a member of the Joint Committee on Accreditation of Healthcare Organizations, ask to see that group's review of the home. Ask yourself if you would feel reassured leaving your loved one there.

Visit again. Make a second visit without an appointment, maybe on another day of the week or time of day, so you will meet other staff members. See if your first thoughts are still the same.

Understand. Once you or your relative have made a choice, be sure to understand the facility's contract and payment plan. If you don't understand it, you could have a lawyer look them over before signing.

How to Pay

There are several ways to pay for nursing facility care for people over age 65. They are:

- Medicare,
- Private pay,
- Medicaid, or
- Long-term care insurance.

Let's see what happened after Alice left the hospital. She went directly to a skilled nursing facility. It had a rehabilitation unit where she began to receive physical therapy. *Medicare* covered most of her costs for the first few weeks as she got better. Then she had a stroke which left her unable to move her left arm and leg. While she was in the hospital for the stroke, her doctors decided Alice should probably not return home. She no longer qualified for Medicare to pay for her nursing home care.

- Many people believe that Medicare will pay for long stays in a nursing home, but it doesn't. The Federal Medicare program and private "Medigap" (Medicare supplemental) insurance only cover short times of home health or nursing home care. They pay for a short stay in a nursing home for someone who is getting better after leaving the hospital, but still needs nursing care and therapy.

Alice's husband started to pay for her care on his own, but they didn't have a lot of savings. When they had used most of their savings, her husband arranged for her to apply for *Medicaid*. The good news about Medicaid is that her husband did not have to sell their home for her to qualify for this support.

- Many people start paying for long-term care with their own money (private pay). Later they may become eligible for state-run Medicaid. Each state decides who qualifies for this program. Contact your state government to learn more. Keep in mind that applying for Medicaid takes at least three months.

Alice's children are now looking into buying long-term care insurance for themselves. They don't want to have the same worries if they need nursing care when they are older.

- Long-term care insurance is a private insurance policy you can buy years before you think you might need it. Each policy is different. Your state's insurance commission can tell you more about private long-term care policies. They can also offer tips on how to buy long-term care insurance. These agencies are listed in your telephone book, under "Government."

Help in Planning

Planning for long-term care is not easy. People's needs change over time. So do the rules about programs and benefits. What someone qualifies for may change from one year to the next. There is some help. The following resources are online. If you or your relative don't have a computer, there may be one at your local library or senior center.

Care Planner from Medicare is online at www.careplanner.org. It has details about different care options. You can answer questions online about needs and resources to get a list of suggested services, as well as helpful resources.

Medicare has two resources on its website, www.medicare.gov, which may be useful. First, *Nursing Home Compare* helps you learn more about nursing homes you may be interested in. They also have a nursing home checklist with tips to use when visiting homes. Second, many states have *State Health Insurance Counseling and Assistance Programs (SHIPS)*. These programs can help you choose the health care plan that is right for you and your family.

Making a Smooth Transition

Moving to a care facility can be a big change for the whole family. Some facilities or community groups have a social worker who can help you prepare for the change. Allow some time to adjust after the move has taken place.

Regular visits by family and friends can make this move easier. This reassures and comforts the person getting used to a new place. Visits are good, too, for keeping an eye on the care that is being given. They also help family to develop a good relationship with the staff caring for their loved one.

For More Information

Other sources of information on long-term care and other issues of interest to older people include:

FirstGov for Seniors
www.seniors.gov

American Association of Homes and Services for the Aging
2519 Connecticut Avenue, NW
Washington, DC 20008
202-783-2242
www.aahsa.org

Assisted Living Federation of America
11200 Waples Mill Road
Suite 150
Fairfax, VA 22030
703-691-8100
www.alfa.org

Continuing Care Accreditation Commission
1730 Rhode Island Avenue, NW
Suite 209
Washington, DC 20036
866-888-1122
www.carf.org

Alzheimer's Disease Education and Referral Center (ADEAR)
P.O. Box 8250
Silver Spring, MD 20907-8250
800-438-4380 (toll-free)
www.alzheimers.org

For more information about health and aging, contact:

National Institute on Aging Information Center
P.O. Box 8057
Gaithersburg, MD 20898-8057
800-222-2225 (toll-free)
800-222-4225 (TTY/toll-free)

- To order publications (in English or Spanish) online, visit *www.niapublications.org*.

- The National Institute on Aging website is *www.nia.nih.gov*.

- Visit NIHSeniorHealth.gov (*www.nihseniorhealth.gov*), a senior-friendly website from the National Institute on Aging and the National Library of Medicine. This simple-to-use website features popular health topics for older adults. It has large type and a "talking" function that reads the text out loud.

September 2003

Older Drivers

At age 75, Sheila thinks she's a very good driver. And she wanted to stay that way. So she got her eyes and hearing checked to make sure she can see and hear well enough to drive safely. Then she signed up to take a driving course for older drivers at her local automobile club. Will all this effort guarantee Sheila's road safety?

As he was driving to the grocery store one day, 80-year-old Daniel ran over the curb and hit a trash can. His car was only scratched, and he was not hurt. But Daniel was scared because he almost hit a young woman waiting at the bus stop. He began to wonder if he should give up his driver's license. How will Daniel know when it's time for him to stop driving?

How Does Age Affect Driving?

More and more older drivers are on the roads these days. It's important to know that getting older doesn't automatically turn people into bad drivers. Many of us continue to be good, safe drivers as we age. But there are changes that can affect driving skills as we age.

Changes to our Bodies. Over time your joints may get stiff and your muscles weaken. It can be harder to move your head to look back, quickly turn the steering wheel, or safely hit the brakes.

Your eyesight and hearing may change, too. As you get older, you need more light to see things. Also, glare from the sun, oncoming headlights, or other street lights may trouble you more than before. The area you can see around you (called peripheral vision) may become narrower. The vision problems from eye diseases such as cataracts, macular degeneration, or glaucoma can also affect your driving ability.

You may also find that your reflexes are getting slower. Or, your attention span may shorten. Maybe it's harder for you to do two things at once. These are all normal changes, but they can affect your driving skills.

Some older people have conditions like Alzheimer's disease (AD) that change their thinking and behavior. People with AD may forget familiar routes or even how to drive safely. They become more likely to make driving mistakes, and they have more "close calls" than other drivers. However, people in the early stages of AD may be able to keep driving for a while. Caregivers should watch their driving over time. As the disease worsens, it will affect driving ability. Doctors can help you decide whether it's safe for the person with AD to keep driving.

Other Health Changes. While health problems can affect driving at any age, some occur more often as we get older. For example, arthritis, Parkinson's disease, and diabetes may make it harder to drive. People who are depressed may become distracted while driving. The effects of a stroke or even lack of sleep can also cause driving problems. Devices such as an automatic defibrillator or pacemaker might cause an irregular heartbeat or dizziness, which can make driving dangerous.

Medicine Side Effects. Some medicines can make it harder for you to drive safely. These medicines include sleep aids, anti-depression drugs, antihistamines for allergies and colds, strong pain killers, and diabetes medications. If you take one or more of these or other medicines, talk to your doctor about how they might affect your driving.

Am I a Safe Driver?

Maybe you already know of some driving situations that are hard for you—nights, highways, rush hours, or bad weather. If so, try to change your driving habits to avoid them. Other hints? Older drivers are most at risk when yielding the right of way, turning (especially making left turns), changing lanes, passing, and using expressway ramps. Pay special attention at those times.

Is it Time to Give Up Driving?

We all age differently. For this reason, there is no way to say what age should be the upper limit for driving. So, how do you know if you should stop driving? To help you decide, ask:

- Do other drivers often honk at me?
- Have I had some accidents, even "fender benders"?
- Do I get lost, even on roads I know?
- Do cars or people walking seem to appear out of nowhere?
- Have family, friends, or my doctor said they are worried about my driving?
- Am I driving less these days because I am not as sure about my driving as I used to be?

If you answered yes to any of these questions, you should think seriously about whether or not you are still a safe driver. If you answered no to all these questions, don't forget to have your eyes and ears checked regularly. Talk to your doctor about any changes to your health that could affect your ability to drive safely.

How Will I Get Around?

You can stay active and do the things you like to do, even if you decide to give up driving. There may be more options for getting around than you think. Some areas offer low-cost bus or taxi service for older people. Some also have carpools or other transportation on request. Religious and civic groups sometimes have volunteers who take seniors where they want to go. Your local Area Agency on Aging has information about transportation services in your area.

If you do not have these services where you live, look into taking taxis. Too expensive, you think? Well, think about this: the AAA now estimates that the average cost of owning and running a car is about $6,420 a year. So, by giving up your car, you might have as much as $123 a week to use for taxis, buses, or to buy gas for friends and relatives who can drive you!

Smart Driving Tips

Planning before you leave:
- Plan to drive on streets you know.
- Limit your trips to places that are easy to get to and close to home.
- Take routes that let you avoid risky spots like ramps and left turns.
- Add extra time for travel if driving conditions are bad.
- Don't drive when you are stressed or tired.

While you are driving:
- Always wear your seat belt.
- Stay off the cell phone.
- Avoid distractions such as listening to the radio or having conversations.
- Leave a big space, at least two car lengths, between your car and the one in front of you. If you are driving at higher speeds or if the weather is bad, leave even more space between you and the next car.
- Make sure there is enough space behind you. (Hint: if someone follows you too closely, slow down so that the person will pass you.)
- Use your rear window defroster to keep the back window clear at all times.
- Keep your headlights on at all times.

Car safety:
- Drive a car with features that make driving easier, such as power steering, power brakes, automatic transmission, and large mirrors.
- Drive a car with air bags.
- Check your windshield wiper blades often and replace them when needed.
- Keep your headlights clean and aligned.
- Think about getting hand controls for the accelerator and brakes if you have leg problems.

Driving skills:
- Take a driving refresher class every few years. (Hint: Some car insurance companies lower your bill when you pass this type of class. Check with AARP, AAA, or local private driving schools to find a class near you.)

For More Information

The organizations listed below offer more information about some of the topics mentioned in this fact sheet:

AARP
601 E Street, NW
Washington, DC 20049
202-434-2277
800-424-3410 (toll-free)
www.aarp.org/drive

AAA Foundation for Traffic Safety
607 14th Street, NW
Suite 201
Washington, DC 20005
202-638-5944
www.seniordrivers.org

The booklet *At the Crossroads: A Guide to Alzheimer's Disease, Dementia and Driving* is available in English and Spanish and online. For a free copy, contact:

The Hartford
Hartford Plaza
690 Asylum Avenue
Hartford, CT 06115
860-547-5000
www.thehartford.com/alzheimers

National Highway Traffic Safety Administration
400 Seventh Street, SW
Washington, DC 20590
888-327-4236 (toll-free)
www.nhtsa.dot.gov

For more information about health and aging, contact:

National Institute on Aging Information Center
P.O. Box 8057
Gaithersburg, MD 20898-8057
800-222-2225 (toll-free)
800-222-4225 (TTY/toll-free)

- To order publications (in English or Spanish) online, visit *www.niapublications.org*.
- The National Institute on Aging website is *www.nia.nih.gov*.
- Visit NIHSeniorHealth.gov (*www.nihseniorhealth.gov*), a senior-friendly website from the National Institute on Aging and the National Library of Medicine. This simple-to-use website features popular health topics for older adults. It has large type and a "talking" function that reads the text out loud.

June 2004

Preventing Falls and Fractures

A simple fall can change your life. Just ask any of the thousands of older men and women who fall each year and break (also called fracture) a bone.

Getting older can bring lots of changes. Sight, hearing, muscle strength, coordination and reflexes aren't what they once were. Balance can be affected by diabetes and heart disease, or by problems with your circulation, thyroid, or nervous system. Some medicines can cause dizziness. Any of these things can make a fall more likely.

Then there's osteoporosis—a disease that makes bones thin and likely to break easily. Osteoporosis is a major reason for broken bones in women past menopause. It also affects older men. When your bones are fragile, even a minor fall can cause one or more bones to break. Although people with osteoporosis must be very careful to avoid falls, all of us need to take extra care as we get older.

A broken bone may not sound so terrible. After all, it will heal, right? But as we get older, a break can be the start of more serious problems. The good news is that there are simple things you can do to help prevent most falls.

Take the Right Steps

Falls and accidents seldom "just happen." The more you take care of your overall health and well-being, the more likely you'll be to lower your chances of falling. Here are a few hints:

- Ask your doctor about a special test—called a bone mineral density test—that tells how strong your bones are. If need be, your doctor can prescribe new medications that will help make your bones stronger and harder to break.

- Talk with your doctor and plan an exercise program that is right for you. Regular exercise helps keep you strong and improves muscle tone. It also helps keep your joints, tendons, and ligaments flexible. Mild weight-bearing exercise—such as walking, climbing stairs—may even slow bone loss from osteoporosis.

- Have your vision and hearing tested often. Even small changes in sight and hearing can make you less stable. So, for example, if your doctor orders new eyeglasses, take time to get used to them, and always wear them when you should, or if you need a hearing aid, be sure it fits well.

- Find out about the possible side effects of medicines you take. Some medicines might affect your coordination or balance. If so, ask your doctor or pharmacist what you can do to lessen your chance of falling.

- Limit the amount of alcohol you drink. Even a small amount can affect your balance and reflexes.

- Always stand up slowly after eating, lying down, or resting. Getting up too quickly can cause your blood pressure to drop, which can make you feel faint.

- Don't let your home get too cold or too hot. It can make you dizzy. In the summer—if your home is not air-conditioned—keep cool with an electric fan, drink lots of liquids, and limit exercise. In the winter, keep the nighttime temperature at 65°F or warmer.

- Use a cane, walking stick, or walker to help you feel steadier when you walk. This is very important when you're walking in areas you don't know well or in places where the walkways are uneven. And be very careful when walking on wet or icy surfaces. They can be very slippery! Try to have sand or salt spread on icy areas.

- Wear rubber-soled, low-heeled shoes that fully support your feet. Wearing only socks or shoes with smooth soles on stairs or waxed floors can be unsafe.

- Hold the handrails when you use the stairs. If you must carry something while you're going up or down, hold it in one hand and use the handrail with the other.

- Don't take chances. Stay away from a freshly washed floor. And don't stand on a chair or table to reach something that's too high—use a "reach stick" instead. Reach sticks are special grabbing tools that you can buy at many hardware or most medical supply stores.

- Find out about buying a home monitoring system service. Usually, you wear a button on a chain around your neck. If you fall or need emergency help, you just push the button to alert the service. Emergency staff is then sent to your home. You can find local "medical alarm" services in your yellow pages.

Most medical insurance companies and Medicare do not cover items like home monitoring systems and reach sticks. So be sure to ask about cost. You will probably have to pay for them yourself.

Make Your Home Safe

You can help prevent falls by making changes to unsafe areas in your home.

In stairways, hallways, and pathways:

- Make sure there is good lighting with light switches at the top and bottom of the stairs.

- Keep areas where you walk tidy.

- Check that all carpets are fixed firmly to the floor so they won't slip. Put no-slip strips on tile and wooden floors. You can buy these strips at the hardware store.

- Have handrails on both sides of all stairs—from top to bottom—and be sure they're tightly fastened.

In bathrooms and powder rooms:

- Mount grab bars near toilets and on both the inside and outside of your tub and shower.

- Place non-skid mats, strips, or carpet on all surfaces that may get wet.

- Keep night lights on.

PREVENTING FALLS AND FRACTURES   **185**

In your bedroom:

- Put night lights and light switches close to your bed.
- Keep your telephone near your bed.

In other living areas:

- Keep electric cords and telephone wires near walls and away from walking paths.
- Tack down all carpets and area rugs firmly to the floor.
- Arrange your furniture (especially low coffee tables) and other objects so they are not in your way when you walk.
- Make sure your sofas and chairs are a good height for you, so that you can get into and out of them easily.

For More Information

Many states and local areas have education and/or home modification programs to help older people prevent falls. Check with your local government's health department or division of elder affairs to see if there is a program in your area:

For more complete information on simple, inexpensive repairs and changes that would make your home safer, contact the U.S. Consumer Product Safety Commission at the address below. Ask for a free copy of the booklet, *Home Safety Checklist for Older Consumers.*

U.S. Consumer Product Safety Commission
Washington, DC 20207
800-638-2772 (toll-free)
800-638-8270 (TTY/toll-free)
www.cpsc.gov

National Center for Injury Prevention and Control
Centers for Disease Control and Prevention
Mailstop K65
4770 Buford Highway, NE
Atlanta, GA 30341-3724
800-311-3435 (toll-free)
www.cdc.gov/ncipc

For more information about health and aging, contact:

National Institute on Aging Information Center
P.O. Box 8057
Gaithersburg, MD 20898-8057
800-222-2225 (toll-free)
800-222-4225 (TTY/toll-free)

- To order publications (in English or Spanish) online, visit www.niapublications.org.
- The National Institute on Aging website is www.nia.nih.gov.
- Visit NIHSeniorHealth.gov (www.nihseniorhealth.gov), a senior-friendly website from the National Institute on Aging and the National Library of Medicine. This simple-to-use website features popular health topics for older adults. It has large type and a "talking" function that reads the text out loud.

June 2004

Appendix

Tips from the National Institute on Aging

188 *There's No Place Like Home—For Growing Old*

194 *Understanding Risk: What Do Those Headlines Really Mean?*

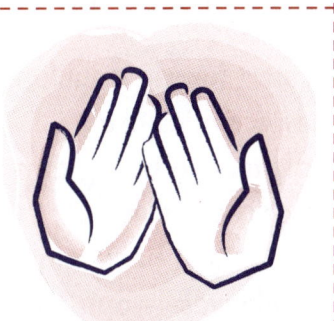

198 *Alzheimer's Disease*

There's No Place Like Home— For Growing Old

Tips from the National Institute on Aging

> "The stairs are getting so hard to climb."
>
> "Since my wife died, I just open a can of soup for dinner."
>
> "I've lived here 40 years. No other place will seem like home."

These are common concerns for older people. And, you may share an often-heard wish—"I want to stay in my own home!" The good news is that with the right help you might be able to do just that.

What Do I Do First?

Think about the kinds of help you might want in the near future. Planning ahead is hard because you never know how your needs might change. Maybe you live alone, so there is no one to help you. Maybe you don't need help right now, but you live with a husband or wife who does. Whatever your situation, start by looking at any illnesses like diabetes, heart disease, or emphysema that you have. Then talk to your doctor about how these health problems could make it hard for you to get around or take care of yourself in the future. Help getting dressed in the morning, fixing a meal, or remembering to take medicine may be all you need to stay at home.

As you read on, you will learn about the kinds of help that you might want to look for where you live. You will read about people and places to go to for more

How Can I Help My Older Relatives Stay in Their Home?

Some people start having trouble doing everyday activities like shopping, cooking, and taking care of their home or themselves as they grow older. Is that happening to any of your relatives—your parents or an aunt or uncle, for example? If so, talk to them about getting help. Offer to get information for them. Think about what you and others in the family can do to help. Talk to your friends whose relatives may be facing the same kinds of problems. Ask about the solutions they found. Then sit down and tell your relatives what you have learned. Together you can decide what to do.

information about the resources near you—from people in your community to the Federal Government. If you are worried about how much this help will cost, you will see that we have tried to give you suggestions for free or low cost help, as well as some that cost more. There are also ways to find out if there are any benefits that apply to you. Last, there is a list of groups to contact for more detailed answers to your questions. Share this information with others in your family, and use it as a stepping stone to begin talking about your needs—now and in the future.

What Kinds of Help Can I Get?

You can get almost any type of help you want in your home—often for a cost. The following list includes the most common things people need. You can get more information on many of these services from your local *Area Agency on Aging*, local and State *offices on aging* or *social services*, *tribal organization*, or nearby *senior centers*.

Personal care. Is bathing, washing your hair, or dressing getting harder to do? Maybe a relative or friend could help you. Or, you could hire someone trained to help you for a short time each day.

Homemaking. Do you need help with chores like housecleaning, yard work, grocery shopping, or laundry? Some grocery stores and drug stores will take your order over the phone and bring the items to your home. There are cleaning services you can hire, or maybe someone you know has a housekeeper to suggest. Some housekeepers will help with laundry. Some drycleaners will pick up and deliver your clothes.

Meals. Tired of cooking every day or of eating alone? Maybe you could share cooking with a friend a few times a week or have a potluck dinner with a group of friends. Sometimes meals are served at a nearby senior center, church, or synagogue. Eating out may give you a chance to visit with others. Is it hard for you to get out? Ask someone you know to bring you a healthy meal a few times a week. Also, programs like Meals on Wheels bring hot meals into your home.

Money management. Are you paying bills late or not at all because it's tiring or hard to keep track of them? Are doctors' bills and health insurance claim forms confusing? Ask a trusted relative to lend a hand. If that's not possible, volunteers, financial counselors, or geriatric care managers can help. Just make sure you get the name from a trustworthy source, like your local Area Agency on Aging. Would you like to lighten the load of paying bills yourself? Talk with someone at your bank. You might also be able to have regular bills, like utilities and rent or mortgage, paid directly from your checking account.

Health care. Do you forget to take your medicine? There are devices available to remind you when it is time to take it. Have you just gotten out of the hospital and still need nursing care at home for a short time? Medicare might pay for a home health aide to come to your home.

Products to make life easier. Is it getting harder to turn a door knob, get out of a chair, or put on your socks? There are things available to make these activities and many of the other things you do during the day easier. The Department of Education provides a website, *www.abledata.com*. If you can't get to or use a computer, they will answer your questions at 800-227-0216. This website has information on more than 30,000 *assistive technology products* designed to make it easier for people with physical limitations to do things for themselves.

Getting around—at home and in town. Are you having trouble walking? Think about getting an electric chair or scooter. These are sometimes covered by Medicare. Do you need someone to go with you to the doctor or shopping? Volunteer escort services may be available. Don't drive a car any longer? Free or lower-priced public transportation and taxis may be offered in your area. Maybe a relative, friend, or neighbor would take you along when they go on errands or do yours for you.

Activities and friends. Are you bored staying at home? Try visiting your local senior center. They offer a variety of activities. You might see some old friends there and meet new people too. Is it hard for you to leave your home? Maybe you would enjoy visits from someone on a regular basis. Volunteers are sometimes available to stop by or call once a week. They can just keep you company, or you can talk about any problems you are having.

Safety. Are you worried about crime in your neighborhood, physical abuse, or losing money as a result of a scam? Talk to your local Area Agency on Aging. Do you live alone and are afraid of becoming sick with no one around to help? You might want to get an emergency alert system. You just push a special button that you wear, and emergency medical personnel are called. A monthly fee is charged.

Care away from home. Do you need care but live with someone who can't stay with you during the day? For example, maybe they work. Adult day care outside the home is sometimes available for older people who need help getting around or caring for themselves. The day care center can even pick you up and bring you home. If your caretaker needs to get away overnight, there are places that will provide more extended temporary respite care.

Housing. Does your home need a few changes to make it easier and safer to live in? Think about things like a ramp at the front door, grab bars in the tub or shower, nonskid floors, more comfortable handles on doors or faucets, and better insulation. Sound expensive? You might be able to get help paying for these changes. Check with your local or State Area Agencies on Aging, housing finance agency, welfare department, community development groups, or the Federal Government (see *For More Information*).

Where Do I Start?

Here are some resources where you can look for this help:

People you know. For many older people, family, friends, and neighbors are the biggest source of help. Talk with those close to you about the best way to get what you need. If you are physically able, think about trading services with a friend or neighbor. One could do the grocery shopping, and the other could cook dinner, for example.

Community and local government resources. Learn about the types of services and care found in your community. Health care providers and social workers may have suggestions. The local Area Agency on Aging, local and State offices on aging or social services, and your tribal organization have lists of services. Look in the phone book under "government." If you belong to a religious group, check with its local offices. The group might have a senior services program.

Geriatric care managers. Specially-trained people known as geriatric care managers can help make your daily life easier. They will work with you to form a long-term care plan and find the right services. They charge for this help, and it probably won't be covered by any insurance plan. Geriatric care managers can be very helpful when family members live far apart. They will check in with you from time to time to make sure your needs haven't changed.

Federal Government sources. There are many resources from the Federal Government where you can start looking for information on help. Some are on the Internet and only available with a computer. Federal Government websites are reliable. If you don't have a computer, you might be able to find one at your local library or senior center. Or ask your local Area Agency on Aging. Perhaps a grandchild, niece, or nephew could search for you. Wherever possible, we have also given a phone number.

The *Eldercare Locator* has information on many different services for older people. They can give you the number of your local Area Agency on Aging. To use this service call 800-677-1116, or go to *www.eldercare.gov* on the Internet.

You can get suggestions to fit your own needs from a Center for Medicare and Medicaid Services (CMS) website at *www.careplanner.org*. You type in information about yourself (age, sex, and whether you live alone, for example) as well as your health problems and other needs. Very quickly it will give the type of help you should look for and general advice on how to find it. The site is also available in Spanish. You do not have to put in any personal information—not even your name or social security number.

The National Library of Medicine's website, *www.medlineplus.gov,* has a section "Home care services." This contains links to information that might be of help.

The National Institute on Aging (NIA) publishes the *Resource Directory for Older People*. It has the names, addresses, phone numbers, and website addresses for more than 260 government agencies, professional associations, and public and private groups that have information or help for older people. You can use it online at *www.niapublications.org*. Or, call 800-222-2225 for help finding the resource you need.

Once you have chosen some service providers, you might be able to get more information about them from *www.medicare.gov*. The *Home Health Compare* section there can tell you more about some of the providers in your state. You can also check on how well these services help people. No computer? Just call 800-MEDICARE (800-633-4227) for the same information.

How Much Will This Cost?

Thinking about how you are going to pay for the help you need is an important part of planning. Some things you want may cost a lot. Others may be free. Some things may be covered by Medicare, private "Medigap" policies or other private health insurance, Medicaid, or long-term care insurance. Some may not. Check with your insurance provider(s). There is a chance that paying for just a few services out of pocket could cost less in the long run than moving into an independent living, assisted living, or long-term care facility. And you will have your wish of still living in your own home.

Once you have thought about which services you need, you can find out about Federal, state, and local government benefits at *www.govbenefits.gov*. If you can't get to a computer, call 800-FED-INFO (800-333-4636) for the same kind of help.

Another website to search for benefits is *www.benefitscheckup.org* from the National Council on Aging. By typing in general information about yourself, you can see a list of possible benefits you might qualify for. You don't have to give your name, address, or social security number in order to use this service.

Are you eligible for veteran's benefits from the Department of Veterans Affairs (VA)? The VA sometimes provides medical care in your home. In some areas they also offer homemaker/home health aide services, adult day health care, and hospice. You can learn more by going to *www.va.gov*, calling the VA Health Care Benefits number, 877-222-8387, or contacting the VA medical center nearest you.

What If I Need More Help?

At some point, support from family, friends, or local programs may not be enough. If you need help on a full-time basis, you might want to think about having someone live in your home. Or, you could have someone from a service come in for as many hours and days as you want for a fee. You might also decide to move to a senior living facility that provides many or all of the services you need. But, in the meantime, you will have enjoyed your home and neighbors for longer than you once thought. A little help from family, friends, and local services will have made that possible.

For More Information

Other resources include:

General Government Sources:

Administration on Aging
Washington, DC 20201
202-619-0724
www.aoa.gov

Department of Veterans Affairs
Veterans Benefits Administration
Veterans Health Administration
810 Vermont Avenue, NW
Washington, DC 20420
www.va.gov

- 800-827-1000 (toll-free) for VA benefits
- 877-222-8387 (toll-free) to speak with a health care benefits counselor

Eldercare Locator
800-677-1116 (toll-free)
www.eldercare.gov

Federal and State Government Benefit Information
800-333-4636 (toll-free)
www.govbenefits.gov

FirstGov for Seniors
www.seniors.gov

Housing information:

Department of Housing and Urban Development
451 Seventh Street, SW
Washington, DC 20410
202-708-1112
202-708-1455 (TTY)
www.hud.gov

Low Income Home Energy Assistance Program (LIHEAP)
National Energy Assistance Referral Hotline (NEAR)
866-674-6327 (toll-free)
www.ncat.org

National Resource Center on Supportive Housing and Home Modification
3715 McClintock Avenue
Los Angeles, CA 90089
213-740-1364
www.homemods.org

Rebuilding Together
1536 Sixteenth Street, NW
Washington, DC 20036-1042
800-473-4229 (toll-free)
www.rebuildingtogether.org

Service providers:

American Association of Homes and Services for the Aging
2519 Connecticut Avenue, NW
Washington, DC 20008
202-783-2242
www.aahsa.org

National Adult Day Services Association
2519 Connecticut Avenue, NW
Washington, DC 20008
800-558-5301 (toll-free)
www.nadsa.org

National Association of Professional Geriatric Care Managers
1604 North Country Club Road
Tucson, AZ 85716
520-881-8008
www.caremanager.org

For more information about health and aging, contact:

National Institute on Aging Information Center
P.O. Box 8057
Gaithersburg, MD 20898-8057
800-222-2225 (toll-free)
800-222-4225 (TTY/toll-free)

- To order publications (in English or Spanish) online, visit www.niapublications.org.
- The National Institute on Aging website is www.nia.nih.gov.
- Visit NIHSeniorHealth.gov (www.nihseniorhealth.gov), a senior-friendly website from the National Institute on Aging and the National Library of Medicine. This simple-to-use website features popular health topics for older adults. It has large type and a "talking" function that reads the text out loud.

July 2004

Understanding Risk: What Do Those Headlines Really Mean?

Tips from the National Institute on Aging

Every day in the newspaper or on television we see stories about new medical findings. Perhaps we hear that a certain drug causes a 300% increase in strokes. That's a large increase—it sounds scary. But, if you know that in every 10,000 people not taking the drug, there are two strokes, then a 300% increase really only means six more strokes. Maybe that's not quite so frightening. It's also confusing that sometimes stories seem to report opposite results—a new vaccine prevents a devastating infection, or it doesn't. How are we to make sense of such stories? How do we know what to believe?

This fact sheet provides some background to help you understand these news reports. It might also help you judge which results are really important and which are simply interesting but not a reason to change how you take care of yourself.

How Does a Research Study Begin?

First, you should know that there are different types of research studies. Often a scientist starts with a question and sets up a controlled experiment to get the answer. Maybe a new drug needs to be tested to see if it cures a bacterial infection. In this kind of experiment the scientist grows the bacteria in the laboratory and then adds the new drug to see what happens. Usually, there is also a *control*—that is, the same bacteria is grown but not exposed to the new drug. The scientist then looks to see how the new drug affected the treated bacteria compared with the untreated bacteria. Perhaps the treated bacteria are dying while the control ones are still growing. That could mean the drug is effective. If so, the scientist might move on to testing the drug in animals and then in people.

Which Studies Involve People?

When studying people, scientists often use *observational* studies. In these, researchers keep track of a group of people for several years without trying to change their lives or provide special treatment. This can help scientists find out who develops a disease, what those people have in common, and how they differ from the group that did not get sick. What they learn can suggest a path for more research. However, observational studies have certain weaknesses. Sometimes differences between groups are caused by something the investigators are not aware of. For any observational study, only further research can prove for sure whether their finding is the actual cause of illness or not.

What Comes Next?

The results of laboratory experiments and observational studies often interrelate. For example, perhaps a new drug for lowering cholesterol has already been tested for safety in a controlled experiment. Scientists know from observational studies that eating a lot of high-fat foods can raise cholesterol levels and they know that people with high cholesterol are more likely to have heart attacks. This might lead scientists to suspect that they can prevent heart attacks by lowering cholesterol levels with the new drug.

But how to prove that this suspicion is correct? Another kind of research study, called a *randomized controlled clinical trial* (RCT), is thought to be the best way to learn whether a certain treatment works or not. A *clinical trial* often involves thousands of human volunteers. They are assigned to two or more study groups by chance (*randomized*). One of the groups, the *control* group, receives a *placebo*. A placebo looks just like the treatment or drug being tested, but actually does nothing.

To start the clinical trial the scientists sign up volunteers. The volunteers are randomly divided into two groups. One receives the test drug, and the other, the control group, gets a placebo. The study is also *masked*. This means that neither the doctors nor the volunteers know who is getting the test treatment or the placebo. For the next several years the investigators keep track of cholesterol levels and heart attacks in each group. They also watch for side effects of the drug. At the end of the study period, everyone learns which group was getting the test drug and which was on placebo, and the results are analyzed. Fewer heart attacks in the group receiving the test drug would show that the drug prevents heart disease.

How Do They Explain the Results?

But, how well does this fictional drug prevent heart attacks? We have to look at how it affects someone's risk of heart attack. By studying large numbers of people, scientists can learn how big these effects are. Benefits and risks can be explained in several ways. These include *relative risk* and *absolute risk*.

When the difference between two groups is described as "relative," it is usually shown as a ratio or a percent. An "absolute" difference is nothing more than a number found by subtraction. How these numbers are presented to you can sway how you "feel" about the finding and affect whether you change your behavior.

Let's look at these differences first by using dollars. We'll compare Chris and Pat's retirement accounts.

	Chris	Pat
Account balance	$130,000	$100,000
Relative difference	30% more than Pat	
Absolute difference	$30,000 more than Pat	

Think about how the numbers make you feel. Would you rather say that "I have 30%

more than Pat" or that "I have $30,000 more than Pat?" Both statements report the same finding, but different people prefer to use different ways to present the results.

If we drop the account balances, would you answer differently?

	Chris	Pat
Relative difference	30% more than Pat	
Absolute difference	$30,000 more than Pat	

Relative Risk

Let's look again at our earlier research example. In describing the results, the scientist might talk about *relative risk*. This compares the likelihood that a person who takes the new medicine will have a heart attack to the likelihood that a person in the placebo group will have one. It tells us how much larger or smaller the chance of heart attack is while using the test drug. Maybe the researchers found the relative risk of heart attack in the placebo group was "1.5." Since a finding of "1.0" means there is an equal chance in each group, the finding of 1.5 means the **chance** of heart attacks in the group receiving the placebo is 50% greater than the **chance** of heart attacks in people taking the test medicine. It does **not** mean half of all those who did not receive the test drug had heart attacks.

Absolute Risk

Absolute risk gives an actual number of health problems that happened or are prevented because of the drug. In our imaginary study of a new cholesterol drug, let's say that there might be 50 heart attacks in 10,000 people taking the drug and 75 heart attacks in a similar group taking the placebo. That is, for every 10,000 people not using it, there would probably be 25 more heart attacks. That's the absolute risk. Some people find absolute risk—"X number of extra cases in 100, 1000, or 10,000 people"— easier to apply to their own health care decisions than a relative risk percentage.

Let's Put "Risk" to Work

How would someone use risk information when talking with his or her doctor about a health problem? Here's an example. Recently Julia learned that she has osteopenia, a loss of bone mass that can develop into osteoporosis. Exercising and getting more calcium and vitamin D are slowing her bone loss. But, her doctor has suggested a drug to prevent further bone loss leading to osteoporosis. Several choices are available. She should ask her physician how well each one would probably lower her chance of breaking a bone as she grows older. The doctor might be able to give her a percentage (relative risk) or the number of times people in the group get sick (absolute risk) for each medicine. Julia also needs to ask the physician about side effects from each medication and her risk of those. With that information, she can take part in making an informed decision about which drug to prevent osteoporosis is best for her to use at this time.

Ask Yourself

So, when you learn about a new medical finding, ask yourself:

1. *Was it a study in the laboratory, in animals, or in people?* The results of research in people are more likely to be meaningful for you.

2. *Does the study include enough people like you?* You should check to see if the people in the study were the same age, sex, education level, income group, and ethnic background as yourself and had the same health concerns.

3. *Was it a randomized controlled clinical trial involving thousands of people?* They are the most expensive to do, but they also give scientists the most reliable results.

4. *Where was the research done?* Scientists at a medical school or large hospital, for example, might be better equipped to conduct complex experiments or have more experience with the topic. Many large clinical trials involve several institutions, but the results may be reported by one coordinating group.

5. *Are the results presented in an easy-to-understand way?* They should use absolute risk, relative risk, or some other easy-to-understand number.

6. *If a new treatment was being tested, were there side effects?* Sometimes the side effects are almost as serious as the disease. Or, they could mean that the drug could worsen a different health problem.

7. *Who paid for the research?* Do those providing support stand to gain financially from positive or negative results? Sometimes the Federal Government or a large foundation contributes funding towards research costs. This means they looked at the plans for the project and decided it was worthy of funding, but they will not make money as a result. If a drug is being tested, the study might be partly or fully paid for by the company that will make and sell the drug.

8. *Who is reporting the results?* Is the newspaper, magazine, or radio or television station a reliable source of medical news? Some large publications and broadcast stations have special science reporters on staff who are trained to interpret medical findings. You might want to talk to your health care provider to help you judge how correct the reports are.

The bottom line is—talk to your doctor. He or she can help you understand the results and what they could mean for your health. Remember that progress in medical research takes many years. The results of one study need to be duplicated by other scientists at different locations before they are accepted as general medical practice. Every step along the research path provides a clue to the final answer—and probably sparks some new questions also.

For More Information For more information on health and aging, please visit *www.nia.nih.gov*, or call the National Institute on Aging Information Center at 800-222-2225 (toll-free).

Alzheimer's Disease

Dementia is a brain disorder that seriously affects a person's ability to carry out daily activities. The most common form of dementia among older people is Alzheimer's disease (AD), which initially involves the parts of the brain that control thought, memory, and language. Although scientists are learning more every day, right now they still do not know what causes AD, and there is no cure.

Scientists think that as many as 4.5 million Americans suffer from AD. The disease usually begins after age 60, and risk goes up with age. While younger people also may get AD, it is much less common. About 5 percent of men and women ages 65 to 74 have AD, and nearly half of those age 85 and older may have the disease. It is important to note, however, that AD is not a normal part of aging.

AD is named after Dr. Alois Alzheimer, a German doctor. In 1906, Dr. Alzheimer noticed changes in the brain tissue of a woman who had died of an unusual mental illness. He found abnormal clumps (now called amyloid plaques) and tangled bundles of fibers (now called neurofibrillary tangles). Today, these plaques and tangles in the brain are considered signs of AD.

Scientists also have found other brain changes in people with AD. Nerve cells die in areas of the brain that are vital to memory and other mental abilities, and connections between nerve cells are disrupted. There also are lower levels of some of the chemicals in the brain that carry messages back and forth between nerve cells. AD may impair thinking and memory by disrupting these messages.

What Causes AD?

Scientists do not yet fully understand what causes AD. There probably is not one single cause, but several factors that affect each person differently. Age is the most important known risk factor for AD. The number of people with the disease doubles every 5 years beyond age 65.

Family history is another risk factor. Scientists believe that genetics may play a role in many AD cases. For example, early-onset familial AD, a rare form of AD that usually occurs between the ages of 30 and 60, is inherited. The more common form of AD is known as late-onset. It occurs later in life, and no obvious inheritance pattern is seen in most families. However, several risk factor genes may interact with each other and with non-genetic factors to cause the disease. The only risk factor gene identified so far for late-onset AD is a gene that makes one form of a protein called apolipoprotein E (ApoE). Everyone has ApoE, which helps carry cholesterol in the blood. Only about 15 percent of people have the form that increases the risk of AD. It is likely that other genes also may increase the risk of AD or protect against AD, but they remain to be discovered.

Scientists still need to learn a lot more about what causes AD. In addition to genetics and ApoE, they are studying education, diet, and environment to learn what role they might play in the development of this disease. Scientists are finding increasing evidence that some of the risk factors for heart disease and stroke, such as high blood pressure, high cholesterol, and low levels of the vitamin folate, may also increase the risk of AD. Evidence for physical, mental, and social activities as protective factors against AD is also increasing.

What Are the Symptoms of AD?

AD begins slowly. At first, the only symptom may be mild forgetfulness, which can be confused with age-related memory change. Most people with mild forgetfulness do not have AD. In the early stage of AD, people may have trouble remembering recent events, activities, or the names of familiar people or things. They may not be able to solve simple math problems. Such difficulties may be a bother, but usually they are not serious enough to cause alarm.

However, as the disease goes on, symptoms are more easily noticed and become serious enough to cause people with AD or their family members to seek medical help. Forgetfulness begins to interfere with daily activities. People in the middle stages of AD may forget how to do simple tasks like brushing their teeth or combing their hair. They can no longer think clearly. They can fail to recognize familiar people and places. They begin to have problems speaking, understanding, reading, or writing. Later on, people with AD may become anxious or aggressive, or wander away from home. Eventually, patients need total care.

How is AD Diagnosed?

An early, accurate diagnosis of AD helps patients and their families plan for the future. It gives them time to discuss care while the patient can still take part in making decisions. Early diagnosis will also offer the best chance to treat the symptoms of the disease.

Today, the only definite way to diagnose AD is to find out whether there are plaques and tangles in brain tissue. To look at brain tissue, however, doctors usually must wait until they do an autopsy, which is an examination of the body done after a person dies. Therefore, doctors can only make a diagnosis of "possible" or "probable" AD while the person is still alive.

At specialized centers, doctors can diagnose AD correctly up to 90 percent of the time. Doctors use several tools to diagnose "probable" AD, including:

- Questions about the person's general health, past medical problems, and ability to carry out daily activities,

- Tests of memory, problem solving, attention, counting, and language,
- Medical tests—such as tests of blood, urine, or spinal fluid, and
- Brain scans.

Sometimes these test results help the doctor find other possible causes of the person's symptoms. For example, thyroid problems, drug reactions, depression, brain tumors, and blood vessel disease in the brain can cause AD-like symptoms. Some of these other conditions can be treated successfully.

How is AD Treated?

AD is a slow disease, starting with mild memory problems and ending with severe brain damage. The course the disease takes and how fast changes occur vary from person to person. On average, AD patients live from 8 to 10 years after they are diagnosed, though some people may live with AD for as many as 20 years.

No treatment can stop AD. However, for some people in the early and middle stages of the disease, the drugs tacrine (Cognex), donepezil (Aricept), rivastigmine (Exelon), or galantamine (Razadyne, previously known as Reminyl) may help prevent some symptoms from becoming worse for a limited time. Another drug, memantine (Namenda), has been approved to treat moderate to severe AD, although it also is limited in its effects. Also, some medicines may help control behavioral symptoms of AD such as sleeplessness, agitation, wandering, anxiety, and depression.

Treating these symptoms often makes patients more comfortable and makes their care easier for caregivers.

New Areas of Research

The National Institute on Aging (NIA), part of the National Institutes of Health (NIH), is the lead Federal agency for AD research. NIA-supported scientists are testing a number of drugs to see if they prevent AD, slow the disease, or help reduce symptoms. Some ideas that seem promising turn out to have little or no benefit when they are carefully studied in a clinical trial. Researchers undertake clinical trials to learn whether treatments that appear promising in observational and animal studies actually are safe and effective in people.

Mild Cognitive Impairment. During the past several years, scientists have focused on a type of memory change called mild cognitive impairment (MCI), which is different from both AD and normal age-related memory change. People with MCI have ongoing memory problems, but they do not have other losses such as confusion, attention problems, and difficulty with language. The NIA-funded Memory Impairment Study compared donepezil (Aricept), vitamin E, or placebo in participants with MCI to see whether the drugs might delay or prevent progression to AD. The study found that the group with MCI taking the drug donepezil were at reduced risk of progressing to AD for the first 18 months of a 3-year study when compared with their counterparts on placebo. The reduced risk of progressing from MCI to a diagnosis of AD among participants on donepezil disappeared after 18 months, and by the end of the study, the probability of progressing to AD was the same in the two groups. Vitamin E had no effect at any time point in the study when compared with placebo.

Neuroimaging. Scientists are finding that damage to parts of the brain involved in memory, such as the hippocampus, can sometimes be seen on brain scans before symptoms of the disease occur. An NIA public-private partnership—the AD Neuroimaging Initiative (ADNI)—is a large study that will determine whether magnetic resonance imaging (MRI) and positron emission tomography (PET) scans, or other imaging or biological markers, can see early AD changes or measure disease progression. The project is designed to help speed clinical trials and find new ways to determine the effectiveness of treatments. For more information on ADNI, call the NIA's Alzheimer's Disease Education and Referral (ADEAR) Center at 800-438-4380, or visit *www.alzheimers.org*.

AD Genetics. The NIA is sponsoring the AD Genetics Study to learn more about risk factor genes for late-onset AD. To participate in this study, families with two or more living siblings diagnosed with AD should contact the National Cell Repository for AD toll-free at 800-526-2839. Information may also be requested through the study's website: *http://ncrad.iu.edu*.

Inflammation. There is evidence that inflammation in the brain may contribute to AD damage. Some studies have suggested that drugs such as nonsteroidal anti-inflammatory drugs (NSAIDs) might help slow the progression of AD, but clinical trials thus far have not demonstrated a benefit from these drugs. A clinical trial studying two of these drugs, rofecoxib (Vioxx) and naproxen (Aleve), showed that they did not delay the progression of AD in people who already have the disease. Another trial, testing whether the NSAIDs celecoxib (Celebrex) and naproxen could prevent AD in healthy older people at risk of the disease, has been suspended. However, investigators are continuing to follow the participants and are examining data regarding possible cardiovascular risk. Researchers are continuing to look for ways to test how other anti-inflammatory drugs might affect the development or progression of AD.

Antioxidants. Several years ago, a clinical trial showed that vitamin E slowed the progress of some consequences of AD by about 7 months. Additional studies are investigating whether antioxidants—vitamins E and C—can slow AD. Another clinical trial is examining whether vitamin E and/or selenium supplements can prevent AD or cognitive decline, and additional studies on other antioxidants are ongoing or being planned.

Ginkgo biloba. Early studies suggested that extracts from the leaves of the ginkgo biloba tree may be of some help in treating AD symptoms. There is no evidence yet that ginkgo biloba will cure or prevent AD, but scientists now are trying to find out in a clinical trial whether ginkgo biloba can delay cognitive decline or prevent dementia in older people.

Estrogen. Some studies have suggested that estrogen used by women to treat the symptoms of menopause also protects the brain. Experts also wondered whether using estrogen could reduce the risk of AD or slow the disease. Clinical trials to test estrogen, however, have not shown that estrogen can slow the progression of already diagnosed AD. And one study found that women over the age of 65 who used estrogen with a progestin were at greater risk of dementia, including AD, and that older women using only estrogen could also increase their chance of developing dementia.

Scientists believe that more research is needed to find out if estrogen may play some role in AD. They would like to know whether starting estrogen therapy around the time of menopause, rather than at age 65 or older, will protect memory or prevent AD.

Participating in Clinical Trials

People with AD, those with MCI, or those with a family history of AD, who want to help scientists test possible treatments may be able to take part in clinical trials. Healthy people also can help scientists learn more about the brain and AD. The NIA maintains the AD Clinical Trials Database, which lists AD clinical trials sponsored by the Federal Government and private companies. To find out more about these studies, contact the NIA's ADEAR Center at 800-438-4380 or visit the ADEAR Center website at *www.alzheimers.org/trials/index.html*. You also can sign up for e-mail alerts on new clinical trials as they are added to the database. Additional clinical trials information is available at *www.clinicaltrials.gov*.

Many of these studies are being done at NIA-supported Alzheimer's Disease Centers located throughout the United States. These centers carry out a wide range of research, including studies of the causes, diagnosis, treatment, and management of AD. To get a list of these centers, contact the ADEAR Center.

Advancing Our Understanding

Scientists have come a long way in their understanding of AD. Findings from years of research have begun to clarify differences between normal age-related memory changes, MCI, and AD. Scientists also have made great progress in defining the changes that take place in the AD brain, which allows them to pinpoint possible targets for treatment.

These advances are the foundation for the NIH Alzheimer's Disease Prevention Initiative, which is designed to:

- Understand why AD occurs and who is at greatest risk of developing it;
- Improve the accuracy of diagnosis and the ability to identify those at risk;
- Discover, develop, and test new treatments;
- Discover treatments for behavioral problems in patients with AD.

Is There Help for Caregivers?

Most often, spouses and other family members provide the day-to-day care for people with AD. As the disease gets worse, people often need more and more care. This can be hard for caregivers and can affect their physical and mental health, family life, job, and finances.

The Alzheimer's Association has chapters nationwide that provide educational programs and support groups for caregivers and family members of people with AD. Contact information for the Alzheimer's Association is listed at the end of this fact sheet.

For More Information

To learn about support groups, services, research centers, getting involved in studies, and publications about AD, contact the following:

Alzheimer's Disease Education and Referral (ADEAR) Center
P.O. Box 8250
Silver Spring, MD 20907-8250
800-438-4380
www.alzheimers.org

- This service of the NIA is funded by the Federal Government. It offers information and publications on diagnosis, treatment, patient care, caregiver needs, long-term care, education and training, and research related to AD. Staff answer telephone, e-mail, and written requests and make referrals to local and national resources.

Alzheimer's Association
225 N. Michigan Avenue,
Suite 1700
Chicago, IL 60611-7633
800-272-3900
www.alz.org

- This nonprofit association supports families and caregivers of patients with AD. Chapters nationwide provide referrals to local resources and services and sponsor support groups and educational programs. The Association also funds research.

Eldercare Locator
800-677-1116
www.eldercare.gov

- This service of the Administration on Aging is funded by the Federal Government. It offers information about and referrals to respite care and other home and community services offered by State and Area Agencies on Aging.

For more information about health and aging, contact:

National Institute on Aging Information Center
P.O. Box 8057
Gaithersburg, MD 20898-8057
800-222-2225 (toll-free)
800-222-4225 (TTY/toll-free)

- To order publications (in English or Spanish) online, visit www.niapublications.org.
- The National Institute on Aging website is www.nia.nih.gov.
- Visit NIHSeniorHealth.gov (www.nihseniorhealth.gov), a senior-friendly website from the National Institute on Aging and the National Library of Medicine. This simple-to-use website features popular health topics for older adults. It has large type and a "talking" function that reads the text out loud.

August 2005

Index

A

Advance directive, 148, 163, 165
AIDS (See HIV/AIDS)
Alcohol, 12, 31, 67, 73-75, 106, 151, 172
Alzheimer's disease, 17, 19, 22-25, 180, 198-203 (See also Dementia)
Anti-aging, 98-103, 142 (See also Life extension)
Arthritis, 4-8, 104, 142-143
Assisted living, 175-179, 192-193

B

Blood, 10, 34, 50-51, 57, 60, 81, 105, 121
   Pressure, 150 (See also Hypertension)
Bone, 4, 40, 44-48, 81, 121, 184
Brain, 22-25, 55, 166

C

Calcium, 41, 44-47, 81
Cancer, 9-12, 41, 50-53, 61, 101, 120-123, 143
   And smoking, 12, 120, 121, 123
   Oral, 127-128
   Skin, 11-12, 116-117
Cold, 53, 170-174
Constipation, 76-78
Crime, 158-161

D

Dementia, 22-25, 183
   Alzheimer's disease, 17, 19, 22-25, 180, 198-203
   Multi-infarct, 22-25
   Vascular, 22-23
Depression, 13-17, 40, 74
Diabetes, 18-21, 34, 59, 71, 105
Diet, 5, 12, 16, 24, 31, 40, 59, 76, 78-83, 91-97, 98-99
Dietary supplements, 7, 31, 79-83, 102
Doctor, finding a new, 134-138
Driving, 180-183, 190
Durable power of attorney for healthcare, 148, 163-165

E

Ears (See Hearing)
Elder abuse, 160
Estrogen, 38-42, 46, 62, 101, 202
Exercise, 6-7, 16, 46, 55, 84-87
   To help you stay healthy, 16, 31, 41, 46, 58, 84-87, 184
Eyes, 18, 20, 58, 69-72

F

Falls, 47, 184-186
Feet, 20, 88-90

Flu, 20, 109, 129-132
Forgetfulness, 22-25
Fractures, 47, 184
Fraud, 142, 155, 159

G
Geriatric care manager, 189, 191
Gout, 4-6
Gums, 20, 125-127

H
Health insurance, 134-136, 140-141, 145-146, 178
Health scams (See Quackery)
Hearing, 26-29
Heart disease, 13, 18, 30-31, 40, 42, 58, 105, 120-121
Heat, 166-169, 173
Herbal supplements, 16, 42, 82, 150
High blood pressure (See Hypertension)
HIV/AIDS, 33-37, 106
Hormone replacement therapy (See Menopausal Hormone Therapy)
Hospital stays, 145-149
Hot flashes, 38-39, 41, 46
Housing/Home, 175-179, 188-193
HRT (See Menopausal Hormone Therapy)
Hypertension, 23-24, 30-32, 40-41, 58, 93-94, 104-105, 120, 167
Hyperthermia, 166-169
Hypothermia, 170-174
Hysterectomy, 38, 105

I
Immunizations (See Shots)
Impotence, 51, 104
Incontinence, 39, 51, 60-63, 105
Influenza (See Flu)

Insomnia, 39-40, 66-68
Internet, 153-156

J
Joint stiffness, 5, 40

L
Legal documents, 162-165
Life extension, 98-103, 142
Living will, 148, 164
Long-term care, 129, 145, 160, 172, 175-179, 192-193
Long-term care insurance, 177-178, 192

M
Mammogram, 10, 41
Medicaid, 140, 177-178, 191-192
Medicare, 9, 20, 129, 134-138, 140-141, 145-146, 164, 177-178, 190-192
Medicine, harmful effects of, 27, 53, 106
    Safe use of, 150-152
Memory, 22-25, 143, 172, 198-203
Men, 10, 44, 47-48, 49-52, 60, 104-108
Menopausal hormone therapy, 41-43, 46-47, 81
Menopause, 38-43, 44-48, 81
Mouth, 125-128

N
Night sweats, 39-41
Nursing home, 129, 145, 160, 172, 176-179
Nutrition, 79-83, 91-97

O
Osteoarthritis (OA), 4-8
Osteopenia, 44
Osteoporosis, 40-41, 44-48, 121, 184
Over-the-counter drugs, 31, 145, 149, 150

P
Pain, 4-8, 9, 49-52, 53-56, 105
Pap test, 10, 41
Parkinson's disease, 172, 181
Perimenopause, 38-43
Pneumococcal disease, 109-110
Pneumonia, 109, 131
Postmenopause, 38-43
Power of attorney, 148, 160, 163-165
Progesterone, 38, 42
Prostate, 10-12, 49-52, 106
Psoriasis, 5, 171

Q
Quackery, quacks, 142-144

R
Rheumatoid arthritis (RA), 4-8
Risk, explanation of, 194-197

S
Sex, 33-36, 39, 49, 51, 104-108
Sexually-transmitted diseases (STDs), 33-37, 39, 106
Shingles, 53-56, 111, 117-118
Shots, 20, 109-113, 130
Skilled nursing facility, 129, 145, 160, 172, 176-179
Skin, 11-12, 20, 40, 53-54, 89, 109-113
Sleep, 14, 39-40, 66-68
Smoking, 12, 24, 38, 40, 46, 48, 58, 67, 114, 120-124
Stroke, 23-24, 57-59, 105
Sun exposure, 114-115, 117-118
Surgery, 11, 29, 50-51, 62, 105-106, 139-141

T
Teeth, 20, 125-128
Testosterone, 48, 50-51, 101
Tests, 9-11, 19, 23, 26, 34, 41, 50, 60
   Scans, 23, 45, 58
Tetanus, 110-111
Tinnitus, 27, 29
Transient ischemic attack (TIA), 57
Trusts, 163

U
Urinary problems, 39, 49-52, 60-63

V
Vaccines (See Shots)
Vitamins and minerals, 12, 16, 31, 40, 79-83

W
Weight, 6, 12, 31, 121
Will, 148, 162-165
Women, 10, 36, 38-43, 44-48, 60-63, 81, 101, 104-108, 121